AAGBI Core Topics in Anaesthesia 2015

AAGBI Core Topics in Anaesthesia 2015

EDITED BY

William Harrop-Griffiths

Imperial College Healthcare NHS Trust
London, UK

Richard Griffiths

Peterborough & Stamford Hospitals NHS Trust
Peterborough, UK

Felicity Plaat

Imperial College Healthcare NHS Trust
London, UK

WILEY Blackwell

This edition first published 2015 © 2015 by The Association of Anaesthetists of Great Britain and Ireland (AAGBI)

Registered office: John Wiley & Sons, Ltd, The Atrium, Southern Gate, Chichester, West Sussex, PO19 8SQ, UK

Editorial offices: 9600 Garsington Road, Oxford, OX4 2DQ, UK
The Atrium, Southern Gate, Chichester, West Sussex, PO19 8SQ, UK
111 River Street, Hoboken, NJ 07030-5774, USA

For details of our global editorial offices, for customer services and for information about how to apply for permission to reuse the copyright material in this book please see our website at www.wiley.com/wiley-blackwell

The right of the author to be identified as the author of this work has been asserted in accordance with the UK Copyright, Designs and Patents Act 1988.

Designations used by companies to distinguish their products are often claimed as trademarks. All brand names and product names used in this book are trade names, service marks, trademarks or registered trademarks of their respective owners. The publisher is not associated with any product or vendor mentioned in this book. It is sold on the understanding that the publisher is not engaged in rendering professional services. If professional advice or other expert assistance is required, the services of a competent professional should be sought.

The contents of this work are intended to further general scientific research, understanding, and discussion only and are not intended and should not be relied upon as recommending or promoting a specific method, diagnosis, or treatment by health science practitioners for any particular patient. The publisher and the author make no representations or warranties with respect to the accuracy or completeness of the contents of this work and specifically disclaim all warranties, including without limitation any implied warranties of fitness for a particular purpose. In view of ongoing research, equipment modifications, changes in governmental regulations, and the constant flow of information relating to the use of medicines, equipment, and devices, the reader is urged to review and evaluate the information provided in the package insert or instructions for each medicine, equipment, or device for, among other things, any changes in the instructions or indication of usage and for added warnings and precautions. Readers should consult with a specialist where appropriate. The fact that an organization or Website is referred to in this work as a citation and/or a potential source of further information does not mean that the author or the publisher endorses the information the organization or Website may provide or recommendations it may make. Further, readers should be aware that Internet Websites listed in this work may have changed or disappeared between when this work was written and when it is read. No warranty may be created or extended by any promotional statements for this work. Neither the publisher nor the author shall be liable for any damages arising herefrom.

Library of Congress Cataloging-in-Publication Data
AAGBI core topics in anaesthesia 2015 / edited by William Harrop-Griffiths, Richard Griffiths, Felicity Plaat.
    p. ; cm.
    Continuation of: AAGBI core topics in anaesthesia / edited by Ian Johnston, William Harrop-Griffiths, Leslie Gemmell. 2012.
    Includes bibliographical references and index.
    ISBN 978-1-118-78087-9 (pbk.)
    I. Harrop-Griffiths, William, editor.   II. Griffiths, Richard, 1960-, editor.   III. Plaat, Felicity, editor.   IV. Association of Anaesthetists of Great Britain and Ireland, issuing body.   V. AAGBI core topics in anaesthesia. Continuation of (work):
    [DNLM: 1. Anesthesia–methods.   2. Anesthesia–contraindications.   3. Surgical Procedures, Operative. WO 200]
    RD81
    617.9′6–dc23   2015016167

A catalogue record for this book is available from the British Library.

Wiley also publishes its books in a variety of electronic formats. Some content that appears in print may not be available in electronic books.

Cover image: Stock photo © knape; from iStock by Getty Images
Cover design by Chris Steer, AAGBI

Set in 9.5/13pt Meridien by Aptara Inc., New Delhi, India
Printed in Singapore by C.O.S. Printers Pte Ltd

1 2015

Contents

List of Contributors, vii

Foreword, ix

1 Abnormalities of Coagulation and Obstetric Anaesthesia, 1
Hilary Swales

2 Acute Coronary Syndromes and Anaesthesia, 15
Yasir Parviz, Rachel Orme, Oliver Watson and Tim Chico

3 Acute Pain Management of Opioid-Tolerant Patients, 28
Mark Jackson

4 Echocardiography and Anaesthesia, 39
Jonathan H. Rosser and Nicholas J. Morgan-Hughes

5 Medico-Legal Aspects of Regional Anaesthesia, 54
William T. Frame

6 Peri-Operative Use of Beta-Blockers: Yes or No?, 65
Nanda Gopal Mandal

7 Transfusion Requirements and the Older Person, 80
Alexa Mannings and Iain Moppett

8 Organ Donation and the Anaesthetist, 91
Dale Gardiner, Neal Beckett, Paul Townsley and Helen Fenner

9 Postoperative Cognitive Dysfunction: Fact or Fiction?, 114
Irwin Foo

10 Pre-Operative Anaemia: Should We Worry?, 127
Robert Kong

List of Contributors

Neal Beckett
Musgrave Park Hospital
Belfast, UK

Tim Chico
Northern General Hospital NHS Foundation
Trust
Sheffield, UK

Helen Fenner
Nottingham University Hospitals NHS Trust
Nottingham, UK

Irwin Foo
Western General Hospital
Edinburgh, UK

William T. Frame
Glasgow Royal Infirmary
Glasgow, UK

Dale Gardiner
NHS Blood and Transplant
Bristol, UK, and
Nottingham University Hospitals NHS Trust
Nottingham, UK

Mark Jackson
Royal Devon and Exeter Hospital
Exeter, UK

Robert Kong
Brighton and Sussex University Hospitals NHS
Trust
Brighton, UK

Nanda Gopal Mandal
Peterborough City Hospital
Peterborough, UK

Alexa Mannings
Sheffield Teaching Hospitals NHS Foundation
Trust
Sheffield, UK

Iain Moppett
University of Nottingham and Nottingham
University Hospitals NHS Trust
Nottingham, UK

Nicholas J. Morgan-Hughes
Northern General Hospital
Sheffield, UK

Rachel Orme
Northern General Hospital NHS Foundation
Trust
Sheffield, UK

Yasir Parviz
Northern General Hospital NHS Foundation
Trust
Sheffield, UK

Jonathan H. Rosser
Northern General Hospital
Sheffield, UK

Hilary Swales
University Hospitals
Southampton, UK

Paul Townsley
Nottingham University Hospitals NHS Trust
Nottingham, UK

Oliver Watson
Northern General Hospital NHS Foundation
Trust
Sheffield, UK

Foreword

Andrew Hartle, President of the AAGBI

Education has been one of the primary objectives of the Association of Anaesthetists of Great Britain & Ireland (AAGBI) throughout the 83 years of its existence. It spends more than £1,000,000 every year supporting teaching activities, and has seen substantial increases in the quality, volume and diversity of its educational output since the introduction of Revalidation in the United Kingdom in 2012.

- *Anaesthesia*, the journal of the AAGBI, promotes academic anaesthesia and education by publishing regular reviews and themed supplements, the last two covering transfusion and bleeding problems, and anaesthesia for the elderly.
- Our online resource, Learn@AAGBI, provides hundreds of hours of videos from the best teachers in the United Kingdom, Ireland and overseas, as well as easy and effective ways to record reflective learning derived from them.
- Our Core Topics meetings held throughout the United Kingdom and Ireland are growing in number, attendance and popularity, with subject areas chosen specifically in response to the needs of our members.

With superb educational material being delivered to our more than 10,000 members both in meetings and electronically, via computers, tablets and smartphones, are the days of the traditionally bound, paper book numbered? To answer this question, the AAGBI published *Core Topics in Anaesthesia 2012*, a collection of eleven clear, concise and up-to-date reviews of key developing areas of clinical practice. The response from our members was dramatic, and the Board of the AAGBI commissioned a second volume of Core Topics articles: *Core Topics in Anaesthesia 2015*. It seems that concise and informative educational reviews presented in paper form are still very much in demand. The reviews in this latest edition cover diverse but critical patient safety topics such as anaemia, obstetric anaesthesia, acute coronary syndromes, postoperative cognitive dysfunction and echocardiography, all written by the leading experts in these fields in the United Kingdom and Ireland. Our readers are the thousands of anaesthetists who deliver ever-safer care to their patients because of advances in clinical care and education.

I am grateful to the authors of the reviews in this book and to its editors, William Harrop-Griffiths, Richard Griffiths and Felicity Plaat. If you enjoy reading it and would like to see more editions of *Core Topics in Anaesthesia*, please tell me by emailing secretariat@aagbi.org with 'Core Topics' in the subject line. The AAGBI, as usual, will respond to its members' requests by delivering what they need to provide the high quality care that their patients deserve.

Enjoy the book!

CHAPTER 1

Abnormalities of Coagulation and Obstetric Anaesthesia

Hilary Swales
University Hospitals, Southampton, UK

Key points

- Abnormal coagulation is a relative contraindication to regional anaesthesia. The risk of neuraxial haematoma formation must be balanced against the risks of general anaesthesia in an obstetric patient – particularly in an emergency situation.
- A history or family history of abnormal bleeding or bruising should be sought from all women. Those with known haematological disorders require optimisation by haematologists and multidisciplinary management.
- The risks associated with epidural catheter insertion apply equally to catheter removal.
- The management of patients with abnormal coagulation should involve senior clinicians.
- If coagulation abnormalities are present, follow-up must be robust to ensure prompt detection and treatment of complications.
- Published guidelines outline the risks of regional techniques in the presence of specific coagulation abnormalities. Guidance for the use of regional techniques in relation to pharmacological thromboprophylaxis or treatment is available. For those with normal platelet function, regional techniques can be performed with platelets as low as $50 \times 10^9 \ L^{-1}$.

Obstetric anaesthetists are frequently required to evaluate patients with coagulation abnormalities who require analgesia or anaesthesia. The management of these patients should be individualised according to the risks to the individual at that time. In addressing risks, those of general anaesthesia in the non-fasted patient should not be forgotten. It is not unusual for obstetric patients to present unexpectedly and out of hours, so optimisation of coagulation and the formulation of a management plan should be undertaken as early as possible in those with abnormalities of coagulation

---

AAGBI Core Topics in Anaesthesia 2015, Edited by William Harrop-Griffiths, Richard Griffiths and Felicity Plaat.
© 2015 The Association of Anaesthetists of Great Britain and Ireland (AAGBI).
Published 2015 by John Wiley & Sons, Ltd.

for any reason. There are several guidelines addressing the use of regional techniques in patients with abnormal coagulation. Since there is a shortage of good quality evidence, these are based largely on case reports and consensus of opinion and, perhaps unsurprisingly, vary widely on their recommendations. The experience of diagnostic lumbar puncture in coagulopathic haematology patients undergoing chemotherapy provides a useful source of data for obstetric patients [1]. The Association of Anaesthetists of Great Britain & Ireland (AAGBI), the Obstetric Anaesthetists' Association (OAA) and Regional Anaesthesia UK (RA-UK) have published a useful guideline that will be referred to in this article [2].

What are the risks?

During pregnancy, aortocaval compression can obstruct venous return, causing distension of the venous plexus within the epidural space and the development of venous collaterals. Venous distension is exacerbated during uterine contractions in labour and both epidural needle insertion and catheter placement are therefore not recommended during a contraction. During routine epidural or spinal anaesthesia, accidental puncture of these veins occurs in 1–18% of patients. If the patient is coagulopathic, the risks of needle or catheter trauma resulting in the development of a spinal or epidural haematoma, which can lead to spinal cord compression and permanent neurological damage if untreated, are increased. Such cases are rare in UK practice, most likely because of the caution exercised by clinicians in the use of regional techniques in patients with abnormal coagulation. The overall risk of the development of a clinically evident haematoma is low. The incidence after epidural techniques is estimated to be in the order of 1:150,000 after epidural placement and 1:220,000 after spinal injection in the general population [2]. It is likely that the incidence is even lower in the obstetric population. Vandermeulen et al. [3] reviewed 61 case reports of haematoma after regional techniques: 41 occurred in patients on heparin or those with abnormal haemostasis, but 15 occurred in patients without known coagulation abnormalities. The review suggested that removal of epidural catheters posed an equal risk to insertion [3]. When low-molecular weight heparin (LMWH) was introduced in the US, approximately 60 spinal haematomas were reported in a 5-year period: a much higher incidence than that reported in the UK and Europe at the time. This was thought to be due to the higher doses and more frequent dosing regime used in the US. The American Society of Regional Anesthesia produced guidelines that suggested a reduction in the dosage frequency in line with European practice, and the incidence then decreased. The use of the newer anticoagulant and antiplatelet drugs is still uncommon in the obstetric population.

One potential difficulty in obstetric practice lies in the early identification and management of epidural haematoma. Women are often discharged from hospital within 24–48 h of regional procedures into community settings. Women and their carers must be made aware that increasing numbness or back pain following regional blockade may indicate the development of a neurological emergency requiring early referral. Referral, imaging and surgery should occur within 18 h for a good chance of full return of neurological function. Any patient with known coagulation abnormalities who has a regional technique must be carefully followed up.

General anaesthesia for parturients with abnormal coagulation

The risks of general anaesthesia, especially in the emergency situation, should always be weighed against the risk of spinal haematoma formation, which can have catastrophic effects but is extremely rare. The reports from the Fourth National Audit Project (NAP4) and CEMACE (formerly CEMACH) highlight these risks. The overall risk of death in those having general anaesthesia for caesarean section was quoted in 2007 as being just over 1:25,000. In addition to the risk of hypoxia and pulmonary aspiration, the uterine relaxant effect of volatile anaesthetics increases the risk of obstetric haemorrhage. If practical, significant coagulopathies should be corrected before general anaesthesia to minimise airway bleeding and decrease the risk of significant surgical bleeding.

What are the causes of coagulation abnormalities in obstetric patients?

The physiological changes of pregnancy affect the coagulation and fibrinolytic systems. The levels of many of the clotting factors increase (in particular factors VII, VIII and fibrinogen) and those of anticoagulation factors decrease, causing augmented coagulation and decreased fibrinolysis. Thromboprophylaxis is increasingly being used in those with known risk factors for venous thrombo-embolism, and women with a history of venous thrombo-embolism are treated with higher doses of heparins. The use of LMWHs has decreased the incidence of heparin-induced thrombocytopaenia but, once given, the anticoagulant effects of LMWHs last longer than those of non-fractionated heparin, and are less easily reversed. This may be a problem if labour starts unexpectedly.

Coagulation disorders occurring during pregnancy and those relevant to pregnancy are summarised in Table 1.1.

Table 1.1 Coagulation abnormalities occurring during pregnancy

Clotting factor abnormalities	
Congenital coagulopathies	Von Willebrand's disease
	Haemophilia and specific factor deficiencies
	Rarer factor deficiencies
Specific obstetric-related coagulopathies	Pre-eclampsia
	Placental abruption
	Intra-uterine fetal death
	Amniotic fluid embolus
	Cholestasis
	Dilutional: major obstetric haemorrhage
	Sepsis
General causes	Anticoagulant therapy
	Disseminated intravascular coagulation
	Liver disease
	Vitamin K deficiency
Platelet abnormalities	
Low platelet numbers	Gestational thrombocytopaenia
	Idiopathic thrombocytopaenic purpura
	HELLP syndrome
	Major obstetric haemorrhage
Poor platelet function	HELLP syndrome

Congenital coagulopathies

Von Willebrand's disease

This is the commonest inherited bleeding disorder. It is found in about 1% of the UK population and has autosomal dominant inheritance, although there is a wide spectrum of severity. It is a disorder affecting the von Willebrand factor (vWF), which is a large protein that promotes platelet adhesion and forms part of the factor VIII complex. There are three types of this disease:

Type 1:	Partial deficiency of vWF but the vWF present functions normally. During pregnancy, there is usually a significant increase in vWF, and levels are often up to the normal range in all but the most severe cases.
Type 2:	In this, there is a qualitative defect in vWF and little improvement during pregnancy. In some individuals termed type 2B, there is an associated thrombocytopaenia.
Type 3:	This is a severe bleeding disorder in which there is a complete absence of vWF and decreased levels of factor VIII. It is unaffected by pregnancy.

Patients with von Willebrand's disease have a prolonged bleeding time and normal platelet count, except in type 2B disease. Desmopressin

(DDAVP) and vWF concentrates are given to increase the levels of vWF, and are most effective in Type 1 disease, in which the vWF is structurally normal.

Although vaginal delivery is considered safe if vWF is >40 IU dL^{-1}, if operative delivery is necessary, a level of >50 IU dL^{-1} is recommended. There is little evidence regarding the safe level for the conduct of regional techniques. Postpartum haemorrhage is a particular risk, as the levels of vWF decrease to pre-pregnancy levels within 24 h. Desmopressin must be used with caution and women must be monitored for signs of hyponatraemia. Those with Type 2B disease should not have DDAVP, as platelet count may decrease further.

Regional anaesthesia is usually considered safe in patients with Type 1 disease, as the levels usually increase to normal levels in pregnancy [4]. The epidural catheter should be removed soon after delivery because of the decline in coagulation factor levels. Central neuraxial block is usually not recommended for women with Type 2 and 3 disease.

Haemophilia

Haemophilias A and B are X-linked disorders resulting from deficiencies of factor VIII and factor IX respectively. Females are usually the carriers of this disease, with one affected chromosome. The clotting factor level activity is likely to be around 50% of normal, but a wide range of values has been reported, and 5% of women have surprisingly low levels due to lyonisation. Haemophilia prolongs activated partial thromboplastin time (APTT). Factor levels should be checked at booking and at 28 and 34 weeks' gestation. The levels of factor VIII and vWF often increase significantly during the second trimester, but there is usually no increase in factor IX levels. Optimisation before delivery for those with haemophilia A requires the administration of a combination of factor VIII concentrates, cryoprecipitate and DDAVP. This therapy may only be effective for 6 h. For haemophilia B, factor IX concentrate and fresh frozen plasma are required, as DDAVP has no effect on factor IX levels. There is a theoretical risk of uterine contractions and hyponatraemia with DDAVP therapy. A plasma level >40 IU dL^{-1} (for both factors) is generally regarded as safe for normal vaginal delivery, and a level >50 IU dL^{-1} for caesarean section. If the factor level is <50 IU dL^{-1}, prophylactic factor supplementation is recommended to maintain levels >50 IU dL^{-1} throughout labour and up to 7 days after delivery. After delivery, factor levels decrease rapidly to pre-pregnancy levels, so the risk of delayed postpartum haemorrhage is increased. Antenatal diagnosis in babies at risk can be performed and, if positive or if not performed, the mode of delivery and the use of fetal blood sampling should be carefully considered.

There is little evidence regarding safe factor levels for regional techniques [4]. Consensus opinion suggests that regional anaesthesia should not normally be undertaken when factor levels are <50 IU dL^{-1} and APTT is abnormal. If the patient presents in labour, there may be insufficient time to perform laboratory tests, but levels taken in the third trimester can be referred to. The epidural catheter should be removed soon after delivery because of the rapid decrease in factor levels after delivery.

Acquired coagulopathies

Disseminated intravascular coagulation

This is an acquired coagulopathy resulting from uncontrolled activation of the coagulation system. This leads to a decrease in clotting factors to a level insufficient to stop further bleeding. Causes of disseminated intravascular coagulation in pregnancy include

- **Placental abruption** Significant bleeding may be concealed, with the only indications being severe abdominal pain and signs of increasing fetal distress. Up to 30% of patients develop a coagulopathy. If the suspected abruption is severe enough to cause significant maternal haemodynamic instability or fetal compromise, general anaesthesia is usually indicated. In cases of suspected abruption without obvious compromise, coagulopathy is less likely and regional techniques can often be used without the need to wait for a coagulation screen, depending on the relative balance of risks. In these cases, tests such as thrombo-elastography (TEG) may prove useful.
- **Intrauterine fetal death** There is an increased risk of coagulopathy, especially after the second week following fetal death. Coagulation abnormalities are present in about 3% of women with apparently uncomplicated intrauterine fetal death, and this increases in the presence of abruption or uterine perforation to about 13% [5]. The onset of coagulopathy is variable but can be rapid.
- **Amniotic fluid embolism** In this obstetric emergency, amniotic fluid is released into the maternal circulation. The cause is unknown but the response is thought to involve both the complement system and the immune response. If women survive the initial cardiorespiratory collapse, uterine relaxation and disseminated intravascular coagulation will contribute to severe haemorrhage, which is often difficult to manage. Diagnosis is by exclusion. Uterine atony should be anticipated, and prophylactic use of uterotonics and surgical methods to increase uterine tone should be employed. Cryoprecipitate infusion should be considered at an early stage.
- **Sepsis**

Pre-eclampsia and HELLP syndrome

Pre-eclampsia is associated with low platelet levels. There is increased destruction of platelets resulting from immunological mechanisms. In HELLP (haemolysis, elevated liver enzymes, low platelets) syndrome, platelet numbers decrease rapidly and liver dysfunction contributes further to coagulopathy. In pre-eclampsia, a decreasing platelet count may be associated with abnormal platelet function and other coagulation abnormalities, and the course is often unpredictable.

Liver disease

Any cause of liver disease can be coincidental with pregnancy and result in abnormal coagulation. Specific conditions of concern occurring in the pregnant population include:

- **Acute fatty liver of pregnancy**
- **Cholestasis** In obstetric cholestasis, coagulopathy may develop as a result of decreased absorption of vitamin K, which is required for activation of clotting factors. Bacq et al. showed that 8% of women with cholestasis have a prolonged prothrombin time but some question the importance of checking clotting in all cases [6]. It is important to check coagulation before regional blockade, but changes do not occur rapidly and are responsive to vitamin K treatment.
- **HELLP syndrome**

Platelet abnormalities

- **Gestational thrombocytopaenia** Platelet numbers decrease during normal pregnancy, but in the majority of women they remain $>150 \times 10^9 \text{ L}^{-1}$, the threshold below which haematologists define thrombocytopaenia. Gestational thrombocytopaenia occurs in 5–8% of pregnant women, usually presenting in the third trimester, but it should only be labelled as such after excluding other causes. The majority have platelet counts between 100 and $150 \times 10^9 \text{ L}^{-1}$ but in about 0.5% of women they are below that level. The decrease is thought to be due to a combination of haemodilution and increased destruction. The decrease in platelet numbers is thought to be balanced by enhanced platelet activity during pregnancy, but in clinical practice it is difficult to evaluate this precisely.
- **Idiopathic (autoimmune) thrombocytopenic purpura (ITP)** This is an immunological disorder that commonly occurs in young females. Some patients will become pregnant in the knowledge that they have ITP, and others may be diagnosed in the first trimester. Platelet autoantibodies are present on the platelet membrane and platelets are destroyed in the reticulo-endothelial system. The production of new platelets

does not match the destruction of old platelets and therefore thrombocytopaenia occurs. Platelet counts are usually in the order of 50–75 × 10^9 L^{-1}. Patients may well have no symptoms but some will have an increased incidence of bruising and epistaxis. There is transplacental transfer of antiplatelet antibodies, so the neonate may develop thrombocytopaenia, which may have implications for the mode of delivery. Treatment aims at increasing platelet count if it decreases to <50 × 10^9 L^{-1}, and high-dose corticosteroids or high-dose intravenous immunoglobulin can be given before regional techniques. Splenectomy may occasionally be required and, if it is, can usually be performed laparoscopically during the second trimester.

Which tests for which patients?

There is no evidence to support routine full blood count (FBC) or coagulation tests in women before the performance of a regional block in those who have had
- normal FBC results;
- no bleeding history;
- no signs or symptoms of liver disease;
- no signs or symptoms of pre-eclampsia, abruption or clinical signs of disseminated intravascular coagulation;
- no recent anticoagulant treatment.

Regional analgesia or anaesthesia should be administered in a timely fashion and not delayed or avoided while awaiting the results of blood tests in these patients.

Full blood count
- In women with known thrombocytopaenia, an FBC should be checked within 24 h.
- In women with mild to moderate pre-eclampsia, the course of the disease can be unpredictable: it is recommended that an FBC be checked within 6 h of a regional procedure. In addition, coagulation tests should be performed if platelets are <100 × 10^9 L^{-1} or if there is abnormal liver function. In women with severe disease, FBC and clotting should be checked immediately before a procedure, as platelet levels in particular can decline rapidly. Women with pregnancy-induced hypertension alone do not require an FBC before a regional procedure.
- Those who have been on heparin for more than 4 days are at risk of thrombocytopaenia.

Activated partial thromboplastin time ratio and international normalised ratio

- Activated partial thromboplastin time ratio (APTTR) and international normalised ratio (INR) are slightly decreased in late pregnancy. The APTTR is a good screening test for deficiencies of factors VIII, IX, XI and XII, and heparin-induced anticoagulation. The INR tests for deficiencies in II, V, VII, X and fibrinogen.
- In women with obstetric cholestasis, coagulation status should be checked within 24 h of a regional procedure, although in practice changes affecting coagulation do not usually occur rapidly.
- In women on heparin (or warfarin), an FBC and APPTR (or INR for those on warfarin) should be checked immediately before anaesthetic or surgical interventions.
- For those on LMWHs, the assessment of anti-Xa levels to determine bleeding risk is controversial, and in practice takes time, rendering it not particularly useful. Although high anti-Xa levels have been shown to be a good predictor of bleeding risk, lower levels have not been shown to be reassuring.

Thromboelastography

- TEG is now providing useful information about overall coagulation status and, importantly, fibrinogen deficiency in haemorrhage, and has the great advantage of being a point-of-care test that provides results within 15 min, thus enabling decisions to be made on the basis of the results in real time. An early decrease in fibrinogen concentration is a predictor of severe postpartum haemorrhage; prompt management can significantly improve outcome. It has been shown that the ability to provide real time, targeted coagulation management can decrease the need for additional blood and products [7].
- The sensitivity and specificity of TEG results in pregnancy and their exact relationship to the risk of any haematoma development is still being evaluated. An abnormal TEG should usually preclude the use of regional techniques.

Guidance for the use of regional anaesthetic techniques in patients given anticoagulant drugs

The use of anticoagulant drugs in pregnant patients poses significant difficulties in balancing the risk of thrombo-embolic disease with that of the formation of an epidural haematoma following neuraxial blockade [8–10]. The key issues to be addressed are planning when to stop the anticoagulant, or

Table 1.2 Summary of the recommendations from the AAGBI, the OAA and RA-UK guidelines [2] regarding the performance of regional anaesthesia after anticoagulant therapy

Drugs	Recommendations for neuraxial block
Aspirin and non-steroidal anti-inflammatory drugs	Antiplatelet effect of aspirin persists until new platelets are manufactured (at least 7 days), whereas platelet function returns to normal within 3 days after stopping NSAIDs. Central neuraxial block can be safely performed in patients taking these drugs.
Unfractionated heparin	Delay block for 4 h after subcutaneous dose and give >1h after performing a block. Stop intravenous heparin infusion 4 h before block. APTTR should be checked and be normal. Restart intravenous heparin >1 h after performing a block.
Low-molecular weight heparin	Delay block 12 h after prophylactic LMWH. Give LMWH >2 h after performing a block. Wait for 24 h after a therapeutic dose of LMWH is given before performing a block. If a bloody tap, consider delaying next dose for 24 h

NSAIDs, non-steroidal anti-inflammatory drugs; APTTR, activated partial thromboplastin time ratio; LMWH, low-molecular weight heparin.

how long to wait before a regional technique if the routine administration of the drug has not been stopped, planning when the drug can be restarted after a regional technique, and patient follow-up.

Even though there are few firm data to support recommendations, guidelines have been produced by the American Society of Regional Anesthesia, the European Society of Regional Anaesthesia and a number of European countries. There are many differences between them, reflecting differing drugs and dosage regimes. The guidance published by the AAGBI, the OAA and RA-UK was based on expert opinion, case reports, case series, cohort studies and extrapolations from the drug properties and the known half-lives of drugs [2]. Table 1.2 summarises the recommendations from these guidelines regarding recommended performance of regional anaesthesia in patients taking anticoagulant drugs.

Guidance is just that; the ultimate decision to proceed or not proceed with a regional technique after an anticoagulant has been given outside of the recommended time range depends on the individual relative risks compared to delaying the procedure or abandoning in favour of general anaesthesia. The risk of thrombosis also needs to be considered if a drug is stopped for a significant time if the woman has a prolonged latent phase of labour or postpartum haemorrhage.

Risk assessment for the use of regional techniques in women with coagulation abnormalities

Table 1.3 is drawn from the AAGBI, the OAA and RA-UK guidance, and summarises the continuum of risk in performing regional techniques in obstetric patients [2]. It was designed to encompass the very real need to view decision-making in the light of relative risks to an individual. It also needs to be acknowledged that there should be no definitive cut-offs on the basis of exact numbers, as risk is a continuum from normal risk to very high risk. Exact numerical values of tests will differ to some extent within the limits of normal laboratory error.

Guidance for regional techniques in women with low platelets

The risk of performing neuraxial blockade in women with thrombocy-topaenia is guided by case reports, experience from haematological practice and expert consensus opinion. For healthy women with no known obstetric complications, there is considered no increased risk of complications with platelet counts $>100 \times 10^9$ L^{-1} [11]. A count of $>75 \times 10^9$ L^{-1} has been proposed as an adequate level for regional blocks when there are no other risk factors and the count is not decreasing [12]. In pre-eclampsia, a decreasing platelet count may be associated with abnormal platelet function and other coagulation abnormalities, especially when the count is $<100 \times 10^9$ L^{-1}, and a coagulation screen should be performed. If this is normal, it would be reasonable to perform a regional block with platelet counts down to a level of 75×10^9 L^{-1} providing the platelet levels are checked within 6 h of performing the block [13]. The rate of decrease of platelet numbers is very important and, if it is rapid, a sample should be checked immediately before the block.

In ITP and gestational thrombocytopaenia, although there are decreased platelet numbers, the function of these platelets is normal or even enhanced. When the platelet count is $>50 \times 10^9$ L^{-1}, an experienced anaesthetist may be prepared to perform neuraxial blockade, but an individual risk-benefit assessment should be made [1, 12]. It is possible that spinal anaesthesia is safe even when the platelet counts decrease to below this level [1].

Risk of regional techniques in women on LMWHs and aspirin

Daily LMWH and low-dose aspirin are recommended for women with obesity or hypertension. This combination is of greater concern than either drug alone but, provided the LMWH is stopped for >12 h, the platelet count

Table 1.3 Relative risks related to neuraxial blocks in obstetric patients with abnormalities of coagulation

Risk factor	Normal risk	Increased risk	High risk	Very high risk
LMWH – prophylactic dose	>12 h	6–12 h	<6 h	<6 h
LMWH – therapeutic dose	>24 h	12–24 h	6–12 h	
UFH – infusion	Stopped > 4 h and APTTR ≤ 1.4			APTTR above normal range
UFH – prophylactic bolus dose	Last given > 4 h	Last given < 4 h		
NSAID + aspirin	Without LMWH	With LMWH dose 12–24 h	With LMWH dose < 12 h	
Warfarin	INR ≤ 1.4	INR 1.4–1.7	INR 1.7–2.0	INR > 2.0
General anaesthesia	Starved, not in labour, antacids given		Full stomach or in labour	
Pre-eclampsia	Platelets > 100 × 10^9 L^{-1} within 6 h of block	Platelets 75–100 × 10^9 L^{-1} (stable) and normal coagulation tests	Platelets 75–100 × 10^9 L^{-1} (decreasing) and normal coagulation tests	Platelets < 75 × 10^9 L^{-1} or abnormal coagulation tests with indices ≥1.5 or HELLP syndrome
Idiopathic thrombocytopenia	Platelets > 75 × 10^9 L^{-1} within 24 h of block	Platelets 50–75 × 10^9 L^{-1}	Platelets 20–50 × 10^9 L^{-1}	Platelets < 20 × 10^9 L^{-1}
Intra-uterine fetal death	FBC and coagulation tests normal within 6 h of block	No clinical problems but no investigation results available		With abruption or overt sepsis
Cholestasis	INR ≤ 1.4 within 24 h	No other clinical problems but no investigation results available		

LMWH, low-molecular weight heparin; UFH, unfractionated heparin; APTTR, activated partial thromboplastin time; NSAID, non-steroidal anti-inflammatory drug; INR, international normalised ratio.

Source: AAGBI, OAA, RA-UK, 2013 [2].

is $>75 \times 10^9$ L^{-1}, and normal coagulation is confirmed, neuraxial blocks can be performed.

Is the seniority of the anaesthetist an issue?

Some guidelines suggest that an experienced anaesthetist should perform regional blocks in patients with known coagulation abnormalities, as the risk of haematoma is higher after a bloody procedure, and the latter is made more likely by a larger number of attempts at needle insertion and catheter placement. However, the potential benefits deriving from a less experienced anaesthetist performing the block might outweigh the risks of delaying while experienced help arrives or abandoning the regional technique and opting for general anaesthesia.

Which technique should be used?

The incidence of haematoma is greater after epidural techniques than after spinal injections. However, when planning the type of regional anaesthesia to be provided, the length of the obstetric procedure must be considered and thereby the risk of converting to a general anaesthetic.

When should epidural catheters be removed?

It is important to ensure that the guidance in Table 1.3 applies to the removal of epidural catheters as well as their insertion. Here, the risks needed to be balanced against those of leaving the catheter in place. Ideally, the epidural catheter should only be removed after a return to normal coagulation status. After major obstetric haemorrhage or HELLP, it may take several days for values to return to normal or acceptable values. The risks of infection, albeit low, delayed mobilisation and wrong-route drug administration also need to be considered.

What follow-up is required?

Guidelines should be in place for the follow-up of all women after neuraxial block [8]:
- Those with known abnormal coagulation need to be monitored closely, and low concentration of local anaesthetics should be used when feasible for analgesic infusions to allow early detection of neurological abnormalities.
- Neurological observations should be performed every 4 h, and continued for at least 24 h after catheter removal.
- If any significant additional sensory or motor defect develops, the epidural should be stopped if still running, and the patient should be monitored for resolution of the signs and symptoms. If this has not occurred

within 4 h, an urgent magnetic resonance imaging scan should be performed.
- Longer follow-up is indicated for those at high or very high risk.
- Patients and midwives should be aware of the signs and symptoms of spinal haematoma, and be aware of rapid referral pathways if complications develop. Surgery on spinal haematoma should ideally be performed within 8–12 h of the identification of symptoms in order to improve the chances of recovery.

References

1. van Veen JJ, Nokes T, Makris M. The risk of spinal haematoma following neuraxial anaesthesia or lumbar puncture in thrombocytopenic individuals. *British Journal of Haematology* 2010; **148**: 15–25.
2. AAGBI, OAA, RA-UK. Regional anaesthesia and patients with abnormalities of coagulation. *Anaesthesia* 2013; **68**: 966–972.
3. Vandermeulen EP, Van Aken H, Vermylen J. Anticoagulants and spinal-epidural anesthesia. *Anesthesia & Analgesia* 1994; **79**: 1165–1177.
4. Choi S, Brull R. Neuraxial techniques in obstetric and non obstetric patients with common bleeding diatheses. *Anesthesia & Analgesia* 2009; **109**: 648–660.
5. Maslow AD, Breen TW, Sarna MC, Soni AK, Watkins J, Oriol NE. Prevalence of coagulation associated with intrauterine fetal death. *Canadian Journal of Anaesthesia* 1996; **43**: 1237–1243.
6. Bacq Y, Sapey T, Bréchot MC, Pierre F, Fignon A, Dubois F. Intrahepatic cholestasis of pregnancy: a French prospective study. *Hepatology* 1997; **26**: 358–364.
7. Collins NF, Bloor M, McDonnell NJ. Hyperfibrinolysis diagnosed by rotational thromboelastometry in a case of suspected amniotic fluid embolism. *International Journal of Obstetric Anaesthesia* 2013; **22**: 71–75.
8. Butwick AJ, Carvalho B. Neuraxial anesthesia in obstetric patients receiving anticoagulant and antithrombotic drugs. *International Journal of Obstetric Anaesthesia* 2010; **19**: 193–201.
9. Horlocker TT, Wedel DJ, Rowlinson JC, et al. Regional anesthesia in the patient receiving antithrombotic or thrombolytic therapy: American Society of Regional Anesthesia and Pain Medicine Evidence-Based Guidelines (third edition). *Regional Anesthesia and Pain Medicine* 2010; **35**: 64–101.
10. Green L, Machin SJ. Managing anticoagulated patients during neuraxial anaesthesia. *British Journal of Haematology* 2010; **149**: 195–208.
11. Rolbin SH, Abbott D, Musclow E, Papsin F, Lie LM, Freedman J. Epidural anesthesia in pregnant patients with low platelet counts. *Obstetrics and Gynecology* 1988; **71**: 918–920.
12. Douglas MJ. The use of neuraxial anesthesia in parturients with thrombocytopenia: What is an adequate platelet count? In: Halpern SH, Douglas MJ, eds. *Evidence-Based Obstetric Anaesthesia*. Malden, MA: Blackwell, 2005:165–177.
13. Sharma SK, Phillip J, Whitten CW, Padakandla UB, Landers DF. Assessment in changes in coagulation in parturients using thromboelastography. *Anesthesiology* 1999; **90**: 385–390.

CHAPTER 2

Acute Coronary Syndromes and Anaesthesia

Yasir Parviz, Rachel Orme, Oliver Watson and Tim Chico
Northern General Hospital NHS Foundation Trust, Sheffield, UK

Key points

- Not all acute coronary syndromes are caused by atherosclerosis and those encountered by anaesthetists may have pathological differences to those seen in coronary care units.
- An elevated troponin indicates an adverse prognosis and justifies cardiological assessment.
- Our ability to predict individual peri-operative risk is modest and our ability to decrease this is even less.

Acute coronary syndromes (ACSs) present to almost all specialities and have probably been subject to more research and clinical study than any other disease. Despite this, many questions remain unanswered about how to predict, prevent and manage ACSs, both in the general population and especially in the context of anaesthesia. This brief, non-comprehensive and highly subjective review aims to discuss the classification, pathogenesis and treatment of ACSs, with particular regard to peri-operative and critically ill patients, which we hope may be of most interest to anaesthetists.

Definition of acute coronary syndromes

ACS is a broad umbrella term. It attempts to bring order to the plethora of diagnoses referring to diseases that have in common acute interruption of myocardial perfusion. The various and overlapping terms used to subcategorise myocardial infarction (MI) (Q wave, ST elevation, non-ST elevation, full thickness, subendocardial, diaphragmatic, etc.) or impairment of perfusion without evidence of myocyte necrosis (unstable, crescendo or

---

AAGBI Core Topics in Anaesthesia 2015, Edited by William Harrop-Griffiths,
Richard Griffiths and Felicity Plaat.
© 2015 The Association of Anaesthetists of Great Britain and Ireland (AAGBI).
Published 2015 by John Wiley & Sons, Ltd.

accelerated angina) are certainly confusing and often hamper communication. Three subcategories of ACS have emerged: ST elevation MI (STEMI), non-ST elevation MI (NSTEMI) or unstable angina. Although imperfect, these terms have come to imply relatively distinct pathological entities, have somewhat different treatments and confer different prognoses. However, as will become apparent in this review, it is still difficult to restrict oneself to any single system of nomenclature. We will focus particularly on ACS manifesting as MI (both NSTEMI and STEMI), since this is of most clinical importance.

Pathogenesis of acute coronary syndromes

Non-atherosclerotic causes of ACS

Most cases of ACS require atherosclerosis to be present in the coronary artery. However, some rarer causes do not. For example, spontaneous coronary artery dissection is not uncommon, and typically affects young women without risk factors for atherosclerosis, which can mislead with serious consequences. Coronary artery embolisation from sources such as endocarditis or congenital abnormalities of the coronary arteries may also present as ACS. A relatively recently described entity, variously termed takotsubo cardiomyopathy, apical ballooning or broken heart syndrome, refers to cardiac chest pain usually precipitated by severe emotional upset such as bereavement or assault, in association with severe apical left ventricular (LV) hypokinesia on echo or LV angiography, greatly elevated biochemical markers of myocyte necrosis, but unobstructed coronary arteries on angiography. Takotsubo cardiomyopathy is provoked by a surge of catecholamines inducing spasm of the distal left anterior descending artery. The LV impairment, unlike that caused by 'true' MI, tends to recover completely after a few months.

Atherosclerosis, plaque disruption and ACS

Despite the relatively rare causes of ACS mentioned above, it is far more common to see atherosclerosis present as ACS in atypical patients than for ACS to be caused by atypical causes. A cardiologist begins to treat ACS patients younger than themselves towards the end of speciality training, with later years devoted as much towards speculation about one's own coronary anatomy as one's patients'. Atherosclerosis starts early and can progress relatively rapidly: in an autopsy study, 20% of US males aged 30–34 had a stenosis of 40% or greater [1]. Though it is common to visualise atherosclerosis as a gradual and incremental accumulation of plaque, evidence suggests a more stepwise increase in size. During plaque accumulation, the artery remodels outwards to accommodate plaque volume while maintaining lumen diameter (so-called 'Glagovian' remodelling). This means obstruction of blood flow by plaque is a relatively late event and arteries that are angiographically unobstructed may still harbour a large burden of atherosclerosis. For this reason, the phrase 'normal coronary arteries', often used to describe coronary angiograms that only report on lumen diameter, is not ideal since this provides limited insight into actual atherosclerotic burden. Newer imaging techniques such as CT coronary angiography can reveal non-obstructive lesions and identify twice as many plaques as angiography [2], justifying introduction of secondary preventative measures when angiography might be falsely reassuring.

Recent advances in imaging (particularly intravascular ultrasound and optical coherence tomography) have begun to shed light on the *in vivo* morphology of human atherosclerotic plaques. 'Stable' plaques have a thick fibrous cap that walls off the blood from the thrombogenic plaque contents, while 'vulnerable' plaques have a much thinner cap, with greater lipid content. An atherosclerotic plaque alone, even one that induces a high degree of stenosis, seldom spontaneously induces an ACS in the general population, though the peri-operative setting may be different as we discuss below. Some degree of plaque disruption is usually required, either rupture (probably at the site of a thin fibrous cap) or erosion. Postmortem studies in humans who died from non-coronary disease have shown a surprisingly high prevalence of plaque rupture (8.7%). It appears therefore that plaque rupture is common and usually clinically silent. Any degree of plaque disruption is likely to induce some degree of adherent platelet-rich thrombus, but the endogenous fibrinolytic system is capable of preventing this from inducing vessel occlusion or even partial obstruction in the majority of cases. However, in the unlucky minority (which we estimate to be around 1 in 4,350 episodes of plaque rupture, based on the incidence of MI of 225/100,000, compared with plaque rupture prevalence of 8.7%), sufficient thrombus is generated either to obstruct the artery completely (typically inducing a STEMI) or to embolise into the microvasculature (typically inducing an NSTEMI), or cause transient interruption of blood flow but without myocyte death (unstable angina)[3]. Since the majority of ACSs are triggered by rupture of non-flow-limiting plaques, many or most ACSs occur in patients with no preceding symptoms of angina. Testing for ischaemia therefore has only a limited role in predicting future risk of ACS. The introduction of routine angiography in most NSTEMI cases has revealed around 10% with no coronary stenosis present. Although some of these may have suffered non-atherosclerotic causes of ACS, it is likely that many have undergone rupture of an angiographically insignificant plaque with subsequent embolisation or clearance of the thrombus generated. In such patients, CT coronary angiography frequently confirms the presence of non-obstructive plaque in the infarct-related artery [2], supporting the use of antiplatelets, statins and angiotensin converting enzyme (ACE) inhibitors in such patients.

In the hours and days following plaque rupture, a dynamic equilibrium of thrombotic versus fibrinolytic forces compete to determine the outcome of the rupture. Generally, this will be towards resolution without consequences, but at any time (most commonly soon after rupture), the balance can tip towards thrombosis and induce vessel occlusion. This equilibrium leads to many ACSs initially presenting with transient or minor episodes of short-lived chest discomfort (at rest, or on exertion if the thrombus induces a stenosis) in the hours or days before an acute presentation. Thus, a first episode of exertional angina due to stable coronary disease cannot be distinguished from an ACS, which is the driver for establishment of rapid access chest pain assessment clinics.

Who is going to suffer an ACS?

The systemic risk factors that predispose to atherosclerosis and thus MI are well understood at a population level. The INTERHEART study showed 90% of the risk of MI could be explained by nine 'modifiable' factors: cholesterol, blood pressure, diabetes, smoking, obesity, lack of exercise, poor diet, psychosocial factors and alcohol (protective) [4]. A person with all risk factors has a risk of MI 334 times that of someone with none of the risk factors. This was interesting in the face of the enormous efforts spent trying to find genetic variants that confer an increased risk of MI, and our not infrequent encounters with patients suffering accelerated coronary artery disease and a family history strongly suggesting autosomal-dominant inheritance. Since INTERHEART, the advent of genome wide association studies has revealed a large number of genetic variations conferring a small (generally 1.2–1.4 times) increase in risk of MI. Despite these advances, no genetic test has so far shown an improved benefit in quantifying future risk compared with clinical assessments such as the Framingham score, aside from a general family history. A search for rare alleles (that would not be picked up by genome wide association studies) that confer a much greater increase in risk continues, though these may be private to each affected family and thus challenging to detect.

Although the nine risk factors listed above help identify who might suffer an ACS at some point, they do not help us understand why the plaque ruptures when it does. Although formerly this was felt to be a somewhat random 'Act of God', epidemiological association studies have identified a range of activities that may increase the short-term risk of MI. Exercise is a double-edged sword; an individual session of exercise increases the risk of triggering an ACS, although regular exercise reduces risk overall. Lower respiratory tract infections probably double the risk of an ACS during that period and it is speculated that increased inflammatory activity leads to degradation of the fibrous cap of vulnerable plaques. A recent meta-analysis found that although the most effective way to induce MI is to take cocaine (increases risk 24-fold), the greatest population attributable fraction was for traffic exposure, possibly responsible for triggering 7.4% of MIs [5]. This study did not estimate the risk of anaesthesia, and we have found it hard to find data on the risk of ACSs induced by non-cardiac surgery. However, since there were 9,000 peri-operative deaths attributed to cardiovascular disease in the 1999 NCEPOD report and 88,236 deaths attributed to coronary heart disease in the 2008 National Office of Statistics report, it is possible that around 10% of all cardiovascular deaths are peri-operative, and a significant number of these are likely to be due to ACSs (we welcome correction!).

Classification of myocardial infarction: are cardiologists and anaesthetists seeing different types?

An acceptable definition of MI has been surprisingly hard to establish, driven by the ability to detect smaller and smaller amounts of myocyte deaths by serum troponin levels, and the wide variety of contexts in which a typical rise and fall of cardiac markers can be observed. Although the pathology of myocardial cell death due to prolonged ischaemia is well understood, how to define this clinically has been subject to repeated revision, most recently in a third 'Universal Definition' published in 2012 by various cardiological societies [6]. The description above of an ACS driven by plaque disruption appears to be generally correct for 'spontaneous' ACSs that occur in the general population, and is Type 1 MI. The driver for creating subdefinitions of MI has partly been the difficulty of how to label the myocyte damage that frequently occurs during percutaneous coronary intervention (Type 4a) or coronary artery bypass grafting (Type 5) which are clearly somewhat different to spontaneous or Type 1 MI. Type 4b refers to stent thrombosis, which can occur even months after stent implantation, particularly in the case of drug-eluting stents that delay re-endothelialisation. Current recommendations are that patients with coronary stents be given dual antiplatelet therapy (aspirin and a P2Y12 antagonist such as clopidogrel, prasugrel or ticagrelor) for one month in the case of bare metal stents, and a year for drug-eluting stents, with long-term aspirin thereafter in both cases. Withholding either agent significantly increases the risk of stent thrombosis, with obvious implications for timing of non-cardiac surgery. Thirty days after bare metal stent implantation, the incidence of major adverse cardiac events is around 10.5%, falling to around

2.8% after 90 days. For drug-eluting stents, the risk is relatively static in the first year (around 6%), falling to 3.3% thereafter. Unfortunately, the panoply of stent names and types do not obviously indicate which group a particular stent belongs to and any stenting within the previous year is a good indication for cardiological review before non-emergency surgery or in the context of the critically ill patient.

Type 2 MI is probably of most relevance to anaesthetists. This describes 'MI secondary to an ischaemic imbalance' [6] and covers circumstances such as MI induced by severe anaemia or thyrotoxicosis (generally in the context of significant coronary artery disease), but also many cases of peri-operative MI or the frequent troponin rises in critically ill patients in the intensive care unit (ICU). The pathology of Type 2 MI is less clear but appears to be driven by prolonged ischaemia, generally in the face of significant coronary artery disease, rather than plaque disruption, as might be induced by prolonged peri-operative hypotension. It is tempting to consider Type 2 MI as what would happen if a patient with angina were forced to exercise long after onset of chest discomfort, rather than being allowed to halt.

The distinction between Type 1 and Type 2 MI is not simply semantic; the evidence base for treatment of MI comes almost entirely from Type 1 MI, meaning that treatment algorithms used for ACSs may be less well-supported in the form of MI frequently encountered peri-operatively and in the ICU. Conversely, Type 1 MI is not uncommon in these circumstances and there is no clear way of differentiating them clinically. This probably justifies treating both types using similar strategies, though where treatments are associated with higher risk of complications (such as antiplatelet and antithrombotic therapy in a peri-operative setting), it is certainly reasonable to judge on a case-by-case basis rather than adhere strictly to ACS treatment guidelines summarised below. For these reasons, cardiological input is potentially of more use than in spontaneous ACS, despite the grumbling of cardiologists called to review yet another 'troponinitis' in the ICU.

Treatment of acute coronary syndromes in peri-operative and critically ill patients

As discussed, treatment of ACS has been defined in large-scale, randomised trials conducted in patients with spontaneous (Type 1) MI or unstable angina, rather than in peri-operative or critically ill patients. Extensive treatment guidelines have been published [7, 8], and we briefly (and non-comprehensively) summarise these below with discussion of their relevance to anaesthetists.

STEMI

Despite the potential pathological differences between Type 1 and Type 2 MI outlined above, in our experience the peri-operative or critically ill patient with typical and persisting ST elevation on a 12-lead ECG (particularly in association with clinical signs of chest pain or haemodynamic compromise) is little different from spontaneous MI presenting to the coronary care unit, and is generally caused by thrombotic occlusion of a major epicardial coronary artery. The mainstay treatment for such patients in addition to beta-blockade and analgesia is dual antiplatelet therapy administered as soon as possible (via nasogastric tube if necessary) and prompt reperfusion, ideally via primary percutaneous coronary intervention (PPCI) [9]. Clearly, such interventions incur a significant bleeding risk that must be weighed against their benefits, and an individualised approach involving the anaesthetist, cardiologist and surgeon is appropriate. The real-world mortality benefit of reperfusion is difficult to quantify: thrombolytic studies were conducted in an era with fewer adjuvant therapies, and PPCI studies compared this against thrombolysis, making estimation of the benefit of reperfusion versus no reperfusion challenging. However, data from fibrinolysis studies suggest that reperfusion within 2 h (achievable in an in-hospital setting) reduces mortality by 44% [10]. We therefore roughly estimate current STEMI mortality at around 6% with [11], and 9% without, reperfusion by PPCI as a yardstick against which to balance risk/benefit considerations. Haemodynamic compromise, ventricular arrhythmia and evidence of significant LV compromise increase risk and thus the benefit of revascularisation, although in the general STEMI population none of these are required to justify PPCI. Treatment with statins, beta-blockers, and ACE inhibitors should also be introduced alongside reperfusion and have the advantage of proven benefit with limited reason to believe that they would be less effective or more dangerous in the peri-operative or ICU setting [7].

NSTEMI

Unlike STEMI, the diagnosis of NSTEMI is often arrived at several hours after infarction has occurred, based on ECG changes and/or elevation of serum troponin, and can be clinically silent, particularly in the case of ventilated or peri-operative patients. In the general population, dual antiplatelet therapy, anticoagulation with low-molecular weight heparin or direct antithrombins, beta-blockers, statins and ACE inhibitors are all used. As discussed above, a sizeable proportion of NSTEMI in peri-operative or critically ill patients will be caused by Type 2 MI; in these patients plaque disruption and thrombosis may play less of a role. Nevertheless, since underlying coronary disease is likely, immediate treatment with statins, aspirin, and ACE inhibitors seems appropriate for all such patients, since these have proven benefit in stable atherosclerotic coronary disease. We would also tend to recommend dual antiplatelet treatment for at least a month and possibly longer in patients without a bleeding risk much higher than the general population.

Several clinical features are associated with greater risk in ACS and well-validated risk scores exist, the TIMI and GRACE scores being used most widely. The GRACE score uses age, heart rate, blood pressure, plasma creatinine, Killip Class (heart failure), elevation of cardiac markers, presence of ST segment deviation and presentation with cardiac arrest to calculate probability of death, in-hospital MI or death, and 6-month mortality. A higher GRACE risk implies that a relatively greater benefit would be achieved from optimal management, and justifies more aggressive therapy, including revascularisation.

In our experience, most debates about management of NSTEMI in perioperative and critically ill patients revolve around whether or not angiography and subsequent revascularisation is indicated. In the general population, NSTEMI patients at high risk of subsequent events (defined by the GRACE score mentioned above [12]) undergo coronary angiography with a view to PPCI or coronary artery bypass grafting during their admission, based on a number of trials showing a decrease in overall adverse cardiac events. However, these trials may not be applicable to peri-operative or critically ill patients because: (i) the likely benefit of PPCI in ACS is to 'pacify' the ruptured plaque to prevent further thrombotic events; this may not apply to Type 2 MI induced simply by prolonged ischaemia induced by otherwise stable coronary artery disease, (ii) the benefit of either PPCI or coronary artery bypass grafting is likely to be eroded or reversed by factors that increase risk of bleeding, prevalent in this population, and (iii) the presence of other comorbidities may also reduce the prognostic benefit of revascularisation.

Even in the general population, current recommendations are that medical therapy (without angiography) is appropriate for patients with extensive comorbidity, and so withholding angiography in a stable peri-operative or critically ill patient who has suffered a proven NSTEMI is reasonable [13]. However, LV compromise, haemodynamic instability or ongoing ischaemia would provide a strong rationale for revascularisation. Thus, for all patients with a suspected NSTEMI, we recommend prompt institution of medical therapy as above, an echocardiogram and cardiological review.

Unstable angina

Clinically apparent ischaemia without evidence of myocardial necrosis, i.e. a normal troponin level, is seldom brought to our attention clinically in peri-operative or critically ill patients but, when suspected, medical therapy as above should be instituted. Recurrent ischaemia, such as angina at rest or on minimal exertion peri-operatively despite anti-ischaemic therapy, would justify angiography and revascularisation if this can be performed with acceptable risk. However, we find correction of anaemia or other precipitants is often sufficient to stabilise the patient, allowing outpatient cardiology follow-up.

Prediction and prevention of ACS in peri-operative patients

The subject of how to estimate risk of ACS in peri-operative patients, and particularly how to reduce this risk, has been extensively and comprehensively covered elsewhere [14], and we have neither the space nor expertise to do it justice. Therefore, we have simply attempted to give an insight into our own practice given the numerous uncertainties while accepting that this is open to debate and perhaps criticism! We also restrict ourselves to the subject of coronary artery disease, rather than valve or ventricular dysfunction.

Cardiologists are commonly asked to review patients before non-cardiac surgery by anaesthetic colleagues, and we suspect this process is often unsatisfying to all parties. In general, consultations are performed as an outpatient, which in the NHS frequently leads to surgery being postponed for many months, sometimes for reasons such as non-pathological ECG variations. Of such consultations, 40% lead to no alteration in treatment and a general recommendation to proceed with surgery [14]. We therefore strongly recommend mechanisms be put in place for multidisciplinary team-type discussions between anaesthetists and cardiologists, since a large number of such cases could be triaged in a timely fashion based solely on a notes review without the need for face-to-face assessment.

When encountering pre-operative patients, we first determine whether they suffer any cardiac symptoms that warrant investigation or treatment irrespective of forthcoming surgery. With regard to coronary artery disease, this is largely based on exertional breathlessness or chest symptoms (we do not refer to chest pain since many anginal patients deny this, instead describing heaviness or pressure), particularly focusing on the functional capacity. Truly asymptomatic patients are generally at low risk, particularly if they can perform such tasks as mowing the lawn or hillwalking. When patients do have symptoms of stable angina, we enquire if they want these improved and if they would be prepared to undergo invasive investigations to gain such improvement. If not, secondary prevention with aspirin, statins, ACE inhibitors and anti-anginals is often all that is required – and these are generally already prescribed.

In an asymptomatic patient, the most likely cause for concern would be a recent ACS or coronary stenting. Non-cardiac surgery within a year of either ACS or stent implantation is higher risk and best deferred as long as possible – ideally at least until the recommended cessation of dual antiplatelet therapy in favour of aspirin alone. This has the advantage of minimising bleeding risk for the surgery. Any decision about cessation of antiplatelet therapy should involve a cardiologist, preferably the one who performed the PPCI and at least after review of the procedural angiogram and notes, as technical issues may influence the decision.

Where further investigation is required for risk assessment, a resting 12-lead ECG, exercise tolerance test (falling out of favour but still excellent for assessing functional capacity) or a myocardial perfusion (Myoview) scan and an echocardiogram are useful and generally reassuring. To minimise delays, we suggest these be performed before any cardiological review. Although Type 1 MI is often caused by disruption of previously non-obstructive coronary plaques that would not be detectable by such tests, risk of Type 2 MI is likely to be higher in the face of inducible ischaemia.

Although the assessments above provide a general ability to identify patients at most risk of suffering a peri-operative ACS, the question of how to reduce this risk remains unclear despite years of clinical trials and debate. Based on the assessment above, patients with intrusive angina symptoms despite medical therapy should be offered angiography and revascularisation prior to non-cardiac surgery, particularly in the presence of markers of high risk (early inducible ischaemia, extensive perfusion defects on myocardial perfusion scan, significant LV impairment). However, in the absence of symptoms or clinical features that would warrant revascularisation irrespective of forthcoming surgery, routine revascularisation simply to reduce cardiac risk is not justified. This leaves medical therapy as the only potential avenue for reduction of cardiovascular risk. Unfortunately, the results of studies in this area have been inconsistent and recently undermined. Below we discuss the two areas most discussed: peri-operative beta-blockers and statins.

Beta-blockers

The uncertainty surrounding the role of beta-blockers to reduce the risk of peri-operative cardiovascular events typifies many difficulties in the field. There is an attractive hypothesis that beta-blockade might reduce peri-operative MI, perhaps particularly Type 2 MI driven by ischaemia, rather than Type 1, since there is limited evidence to suggest beta-blockers influence plaque rupture. Current guidance (from cardiological societies) continues to support the use of peri-operative beta-blockade in high-risk patients, and in particular that established beta-blockade for existing indications should be continued through the peri-operative period. These recommendations are based on a series of rather small and inconsistent clinical studies [14]. The largest randomised controlled trial, which reported after these guidelines, was the POISE study. This randomised high-risk patients undergoing non-cardiac surgery to receive metoprolol or placebo 2–4 h before surgery. From a cardiological viewpoint, it supported the hypothesis above: beta-blockade did indeed reduce the risk of MI or a composite cardiovascular endpoint. However, this was outweighed by an increase in stroke and overall mortality in the beta-blocker-treated group, dampening enthusiasm for peri-operative beta-blockers. The potential reasons for the POISE findings are legion and unnecessary to rehearse here, aside from noting that both beta-blocker protagonists and antagonists can find much ammunition within its results.

The entire debate has recently been coloured by the dismissal for alleged research misconduct of one of the leading figures in the field, whose work largely supported the use of peri-operative beta-blockade [15]. Although the facts are unclear, this cannot help but throw the subject into even more confusion. Effectively, we are little further on than 20 years ago.

What do we do in the face of this? We continue (perhaps wrongly) to hope that peri-operative beta-blockers, when administered correctly, i.e. not started immediately before surgery, and when well tolerated, may reduce cardiovascular events in high-risk patients undergoing non-cardiac surgery. We still advise against cessation of such agents, and sometimes introduce them weeks before surgery in high-risk patients with evidence of ischaemia and no cerebrovascular or carotid disease. We welcome discussion on this point, but would also suggest that well-conducted registries might be the only way to resolve whether the risks of peri-operative beta-blockers can be minimised while maximising their potential benefits.

Statins

The favourable effect of statins on cardiovascular events is suggested to be mediated by alteration in plaque vulnerability to rupture, rather than reduction in plaque size, which is minimal even with aggressive lipid lowering. It is plausible therefore that statin therapy might reduce the risk of Type 1 MI in the peri-operative period. Observational, case-controlled, or retrospective studies have supported this hypothesis [14], and one randomised controlled trial has shown statin therapy to reduce cardiovascular mortality in patients undergoing vascular surgery [16], although this study is also tainted by suggestions of potential research misconduct [15]. We treat all patients with known coronary artery disease with statins. Regarding peri-operative optimisation, it seems appropriate to ensure that cholesterol levels are to target and that the statin is not discontinued. Extension of statin therapy to patients at high risk of coronary artery disease seems also justifiable, and where a patient may have angina, but this has not been fully investigated. We accept there is an argument for cardiological assessment even when revascularisation is not warranted on symptom levels.

Conclusion

Our understanding of the epidemiology, genetics, pathogenesis and treatment of ACS has made great advances in the last two decades. However, we hope this review serves to underline how much more there is to understand. Given the large number of uncertainties, close communication between anaesthetists and cardiologists is highly desirable in the management of patients suffering or at risk of ACS.

References

1. McGill HC Jr, McMahan CA, Zieske AW, et al. Association of coronary heart disease risk factors with microscopic qualities of coronary atherosclerosis in youth. *Circulation* 2000; **102**: 374–379.
2. Aldrovandi A, Cademartiri F, Arduini D, et al. Computed tomography coronary angiography in patients with acute myocardial infarction without significant coronary stenosis. *Circulation* 2012; **126**: 3000–3007.
3. Davies MJ. The pathophysiology of acute coronary syndromes. *Heart* 2000; **83**: 361–366.
4. Yusuf S, Hawken S, Ounpuu S, et al. Effect of potentially modifiable risk factors associated with myocardial infarction in 52 countries (the INTERHEART study): case-control study. *Lancet* 2004; **364**: 937–952.
5. Nawrot TS, Perez L, Kunzli N, Munters E, Nemery B. Public health importance of triggers of myocardial infarction: a comparative risk assessment. *Lancet* 2011; **377**: 732–740.
6. Thygesen K, Alpert JS, Jaffe AS, et al. Third universal definition of myocardial infarction. *Journal of the American College of Cardiology* 2012; **60**: 1581–1598.
7. O'Gara PT, Kushner FG, Ascheim DD, et al. ACCF/AHA guideline for the management of ST-elevation myocardial infarction: a report of the American College of Cardiology Foundation/American Heart Association Task Force on Practice Guidelines. *Circulation* 2013; **127**: e362–e425.
8. Hamm CW, Bassand JP, Agewall S, et al. ESC guidelines for the management of acute coronary syndromes in patients presenting without persistent ST-segment elevation: the task force for the management of acute coronary syndromes (ACS) in patients presenting without persistent ST-segment elevation of the European Society of Cardiology (ESC). *European Heart Journal* 2011; **32**: 2999–3054.
9. O'Gara PT, Kushner FG, Ascheim DD, et al. ACCF/AHA guideline for the management of ST-elevation myocardial infarction: executive summary: a report of the American College of Cardiology Foundation/American Heart Association Task Force on Practice Guidelines. *Circulation* 2013; **127**: 529–555.
10. Boersma E, Maas AC, Deckers JW, Simoons ML. Early thrombolytic treatment in acute myocardial infarction: reappraisal of the golden hour. *Lancet* 1996; **348**: 771–775.
11. Boden WE, Eagle K, Granger CB. Reperfusion strategies in acute ST-segment elevation myocardial infarction: a comprehensive review of contemporary management options. *Journal of the American College of Cardiology* 2007; **50**: 917–929.

12. Global Registry of Acute Coronary Events. http://www.outcomes-umassmed.org/GRACE/default.aspx (accessed 30/11/2014).

13. Jneid H, Anderson JL, Wright RS, et al. ACCF/AHA focused update of the guideline for the management of patients with unstable angina/non-ST-elevation myocardial infarction (updating the 2007 guideline and replacing the 2011 focused update): a report of the American College of Cardiology Foundation/American Heart Association Task Force on Practice Guidelines. *Circulation* 2012; **126**: 875–910.

14. Fleisher LA, Beckman JA, Brown KA, et al. ACC/AHA 2007 guidelines on perioperative cardiovascular evaluation and care for noncardiac surgery: a report of the American College of Cardiology/American Heart Association Task Force on Practice Guidelines (writing committee to revise the 2002 guidelines on perioperative cardiovascular evaluation for noncardiac surgery). *Circulation* 2007; **116**: e418–e500.

15. Chopra V, Eagle KA. Perioperative mischief: the price of academic misconduct. *American Journal of Medicine* 2012; **125**: 953–955.

16. Schouten O, Boersma E, Hoeks SE, et al. Fluvastatin and perioperative events in patients undergoing vascular surgery. *New England Journal of Medicine* 2009; **361**: 980–989.

CHAPTER 3

Acute Pain Management of Opioid-Tolerant Patients

Mark Jackson

Royal Devon and Exeter Hospital, Exeter, UK

Key points

- Assessment and management of acute pain in opioid-tolerant patients can be challenging and their pain is often poorly managed in the hospital setting.
- The provision of effective analgesia needs to incorporate a plan to manage the patient's opioids so that their usual opioid dose is continued to prevent a withdrawal syndrome, and additional opioids are given for their acute pain.
- Ketamine infusions can decrease pain scores and postoperative opioid usage in opioid-tolerant patients following surgery. Oral gabapentin and intravenous lidocaine infusions may have a role as opioid-sparing adjuncts.
- Opioid conversion tables should be used only as a rough guide when switching from one opioid to another. Having calculated the equi-analgesic dose of the new opioid, it is generally recommended to decrease this dose by 30–50% due to incomplete cross-tolerance between different opioids.
- Be aware of the potential acute pain management problems of patients taking high-dose sublingual buprenorphine.

Opioid-tolerant patients are a group in whom assessment and management of their acute pain is challenging, and this often leads to them being poorly managed in the hospital setting. Compared with opioid-naïve patients, they create a greater workload for healthcare professionals and acute pain teams, as they need frequent review and changes to their prescription and patient-controlled analgesia (PCA) charts, with increased bolus doses and background infusions of PCA opioids. They also have an increased opioid consumption, utilising 2–3 times more opioid via PCA after surgery than their opioid-naïve counterparts. They consistently report higher rest and dynamic pain scores when compared to their opioid-naïve counterparts, which makes their assessment challenging.

AAGBI Core Topics in Anaesthesia 2015, Edited by William Harrop-Griffiths, Richard Griffiths and Felicity Plaat.
© 2015 The Association of Anaesthetists of Great Britain and Ireland (AAGBI).
Published 2015 by John Wiley & Sons, Ltd.

Opioid tolerance is likely to be encountered in specific patients groups:

- Patients who are prescribed long-term opioids for the treatment of either chronic non-cancer pain or cancer pain.
- Patients with a substance abuse disorder with continuing illicit use of opioids, particularly intravenous drug users or patients who are currently on a maintenance treatment program of either methadone or sublingual buprenorphine.
- There is also emerging evidence that acute opioid tolerance can occur over surprisingly short periods of time in response to intravenous administration of high-potency opioids, particularly remifentanil.

There is currently limited high-level evidence to guide the management of this group of patients, and guidelines are largely based on evidence from case studies, case reports and expert consensus. This chapter aims to review the current recommendations relating to this group of patients and will outline the approach to management of acute pain in the opioid-tolerant patient in the hospital setting.

Definitions

It is essential to use consistent definitions to prevent misconceptions and mislabelling of these patients. Healthcare providers should be able to differentiate between the term 'addiction' and the normal physiological consequences of remaining on long-term opioids such as tolerance and physical dependence. Table 3.1 shows the consensus statement for these definitions

Table 3.1 Definitions

Tolerance	A predictable physiological decrease in the effect of a drug over time so that a progressive increase in the amount of that drug is required over time.
Physical dependence	A physiological adaptation to a drug whereby abrupt discontinuation or reversal of that drug, or a sudden reduction in its dose, leads to a withdrawal syndrome.
Addiction	A disease that is characterised by aberrant drug-seeking behaviour and maladaptive drug-taking behaviours that may include cravings, compulsive drug use and loss of control over drug use, despite the risk of physical, social and psychological harm. Unlike tolerance and physical dependence, addiction is not a predictable effect of a drug.
Pseudo-addiction	Behaviours that may seem inappropriately drug-seeking but are the result of under treatment and resolve when pain relief is adequate.

Source: American Academy of Pain Medicine 2001. http://www.asam.org/docs/publicy-policy-statements/1opioid-definitions-consensus-2-011.pdf?sfvrsn=0 (accessed 30/11/2014).

developed by the American Pain Society, the American Academy of Pain Medicine and the American Society of Addiction Medicine.

Opioid-tolerant patients generally fall into four main groups:

1. Patients with chronic non-cancer pain

A recent epidemiological study indicated that the prevalence of moderate to severe chronic non-cancer pain in the UK is 13% [1]. This is a significant worldwide problem and the use of long-term opioid medication to treat it has been increasing over the last two decades. In the UK, the number of prescriptions for opioids in the community has increased from 6,000,000 to 15,000,000 from 1999 to 2008 (NHS Information Centre data). There is increasing debate as to the role that long-term opioids should play in the management of this group of patients, particularly with our increasing knowledge about the risks of endocrine dysfunction and the development of opioid-induced hyperalgesia associated with long-term opioid use. However, long-term opioids still play a major role in the management of this group of patients and are thus frequently encountered during elective and emergency surgery.

2. Patients with persistent cancer pain

Opioids remain the mainstay of initial treatment for both background and breakthrough pain in patients with cancer. Pain is often the first symptom in 25–50% of all patients with cancer and up to 75–95% of patients with advanced disease must cope with persistent pain. Cancer pain may be related to disease progression from local invasion of the primary tumour, from metastases or as a consequence of treatments such as surgery, chemotherapy or localised radiotherapy.

3. Patients with a substance abuse disorder

These patients fall into three distinct subgroups.

 i **Active** – patients who are currently abusing prescribed or non-prescribed opioid medication. Intravenous drug abusers are more likely to present with certain types of acute pain, including traumatic injury, limb ischaemia due to accidental intra-arterial injection and infections such as epidural abscess and infections around injection sites.

 ii **Replacement therapy** – opioid maintenance therapy is increasingly recognised to be an effective management strategy for opioid addiction, with oral methadone the most commonly used drug. The methadone maintenance program is effective in reducing injecting behaviour, illicit drug use, criminal activity and cost to society. High-dose sublingual buprenorphine is being increasingly used as a maintenance therapy in opioid addiction, as it is perceived to have fewer adverse effects and less social stigma than methadone. Buprenorphine is a partial opioid agonist and thus antagonises the effects of additional illicit or therapeutic opioids that are taken. It has a high-opioid receptor affinity: standard doses of supplemental opioids do not readily displace it from opioid receptors, making it ideal for use as maintenance therapy. However, when administered in high doses as part of the maintenance program, the management of acute pain with conventional doses of opioids is difficult. Management of this group of patients will be discussed in detail later.

iii Recovery – patients who are now opioid-free are often concerned that if they are prescribed opioids to manage their acute pain, they will relapse into their previous opioid abuse. Patients should be reassured that the risk of reverting to an active addiction disorder is small; there is no evidence that the use of appropriate doses of opioids to manage their acute pain will increase the risk of relapse.

4. Patients with acute opioid tolerance

There is emerging evidence that opioid tolerance and opioid-induced hyperalgesia can develop over a short period of time. Opioid-induced hyperalgesia has been shown to occur with the administration of long-term opioids, following activation of pronociceptive mechanisms in the central nervous system such as glial cell activation, glutaminergic activation of the n-methyl-d-aspartate (NMDA) receptor and alterations in opioid intracellular signalling. These changes can cause an actual increase in pain sensitivity and, paradoxically, reducing the dose of opioids actually improves analgesia. This has been demonstrated in patients on long-term opioids, particularly those on methadone maintenance. Opioid tolerance and opioid-induced hyperalgesia are also associated with the short-term use of high potency opioids, for example remifentanil, used during surgery. This association has not been fully established and there is conflicting evidence.

Assessment and monitoring

Opioid-tolerant patients consistently report having higher rest and dynamic pain scores, which can make assessment challenging. Often staff need to assess the patients in terms of what they are able to do functionally: ability to cough, breathe deeply, mobilise, and follow physiotherapy exercises, as these are more useful in guiding a pain management treatment plan, rather than relying on pain scores. It is also important to monitor for opioid-related side effects, including respiratory depression, sedation, nausea and vomiting, constipation, pruritus and to monitor for signs of opioid withdrawal (Table 3.2).

Table 3.2 Symptoms and signs of opioid withdrawal

- Sweating
- Feeling hot or cold
- Dilated pupils
- Anorexia
- Abdominal cramps
- Nausea and vomiting
- Diarrhoea
- Insomnia
- Tachycardia and hypertension
- Muscular aches and pains

Aims of acute pain management in opioid-dependent patients

It is important to adhere to a clear and well-documented acute pain management plan that both healthcare staff and patient are fully aware of. The aims of pain management are divided into:

1. The provision of effective analgesia

As with all treatment plans for the management of acute pain, a multimodal approach is recommended. Effective analgesia should incorporate a plan to manage the patient's opioids so that their usual opioid dose is continued and prevents a withdrawal syndrome. Additional opioids are given to treat the acute pain, as is discussed in detail below. It is also important to maximise opioid-sparing techniques.

- Regularly prescribed paracetamol, non-steroidal anti-inflammatory drugs or COX-2 inhibitors should be used unless contraindicated.
- Local anaesthetic techniques should be used where possible: catheter-based techniques allow the continuous infusion of local anaesthetic in the postoperative period, decreasing the amount of additional opioid required.
- Ketamine can decrease pain scores and postoperative opioid use in opioid-tolerant patients after surgery. Ketamine acts primarily as a non-competitive antagonist of NMDA receptors, which are believed to be involved in the development of opioid tolerance and opioid-induced hyperalgesia. Animal studies have indicated that ketamine can attenuate both these phenomena. Ketamine is generally administered in low,

sub-anaesthetic doses as a continuous intravenous or subcutaneous infusion after surgery. Various infusion rates are quoted in the literature but the recommended initial starting rates for adults are 0.1 mg kg^{-1} h^{-1} or 100–200 mg over 24 h. Doses may need to be reduced in the elderly. It is advisable to give ketamine separately at a set rate rather than adding ketamine to the PCA opioid syringe. Opioid-tolerant patients can use two to three times more opioid after surgery than opioid-naïve patients; this could potentially lead to more ketamine-related side effects when a fixed dose of ketamine is added to PCA. A study by Loftus et al. looked at the use of peri-operative ketamine infusions for opioid-dependent patients with chronic back pain undergoing spinal surgery [2]. Intravenous ketamine was given as a bolus dose 0.5 mg kg^{-1} at induction followed by a continuous infusion of 10 µg kg^{-1} min^{-1} until wound closure. Total morphine consumption was significantly reduced in the treatment group at 48 h and average pain intensity scores were significantly decreased immediately after surgery and at 6 weeks after surgery.

- Gabapentinoids (gabapentin and pregabalin) are calcium channel modulators and have an established role in the treatment of neuropathic pain. A number of studies has shown that pre-operative and postoperative gabapentin can lead to improved analgesia and decreased postoperative opioid consumption, but at the cost of increased sedation. These studies were on non-opioid-tolerant patients. However, the gabapentinoids may have a role to play in the difficult-to-manage opioid-tolerant patient as an opioid-sparing adjunct, although there is little clinical evidence to support their use in this group of patients or to guide the dosing regimen. Studies looking at gabapentin and postoperative pain in opioid-naïve patients have used pre-operative doses of 300–1200 mg, with some studies continuing administration for one or two postoperative doses. In opioid-tolerant patients in whom I am considering adding in a gabapentinoid as an opioid-sparing adjunct, I use postoperative doses similar to that for initial management of neuropathic pain, for example gabapentin 100–300 mg three times daily or pregabalin 75 mg twice daily, and titrate according to efficacy and side effects.

- Intravenous lidocaine infusions given peri-operatively for open and laparoscopic abdominal surgery in opioid-naïve patients have resulted in significant decreases in postoperative pain intensity scores and opioid consumption compared to a control group. Interestingly, peri-operative lidocaine infusions have been studied in patients undergoing tonsillectomy, total hip arthroplasty and coronary artery bypass surgery with no improvement in postoperative analgesia. Intravenous lidocaine infusion may have a role as an opioid-sparing adjunct for opioid-tolerant patients undergoing abdominal surgery but there have been no studies as yet looking at its efficacy in this patient group.

2. Prevention of withdrawal and opioid management

It is important to re-emphasise that all opioid-tolerant patients run the risk of suffering withdrawal symptoms (Table 3.2) if their normal dose of opioid is suddenly stopped, the dose reduced too quickly or the effect of the opioid reversed by an antagonist, such as naloxone. This is not a sign that they are addicted to opioids, but is an expected physiological response due to the normal adaptation of physical dependence that occurs in all patients on long-term opioids. When managing a patient's opioid requirements, it is important to consider two aspects: first, to maintain their usual opioid requirements to prevent withdrawal; and second, to give additional immediate release opioid to manage their acute pain.

i) **Continuing the dose of usual opioid to prevent withdrawal.** It is important to continue the patient's usual dose of opioid both before and after surgery. If the patient normally takes oral medication and is nil by mouth, an equivalent parenteral replacement will be needed.

If the patient's normal opioid requirements are provided by transdermal patches (fentanyl or buprenorphine), it is generally recommended that the patches be continued, but care should be taken when using peri-operative patient heating devices, as direct warming of the transdermal patch can speed up drug release. The potency of transdermal patches, and in particular fentanyl, is often underestimated, and removal of these patches without addition of an appropriate dose of another opioid increases the risk of precipitating opioid withdrawal (see Table 3.3 for comparisons of oral morphine and transdermal patch dosage). As buprenorphine is a partial agonist and in sufficient doses can antagonise full opioid agonists, there is concern

Table 3.3 Comparison of oral morphine and transdermal patch dosage

Oral morphine; mg per 24 h	Buprenorphine patch; $\mu g\ h^{-1}$	Fentanyl patch; $\mu g\ h^{-1}$
10	5	
15	10	
30	20	
45		12
60	35	
90	52.5	25
120	70	
180		50
270		75
360		100

Source: Opioids for persistent pain: Good practice. January 2010. The British Pain Society. https://www.britishpainsociety.org (accessed 21/4/2015).

that leaving buprenorphine patches in place may make acute pain management more difficult. However, buprenorphine transdermal patches up to 70 µg h^{-1} are unlikely to interfere with the use of a full opioid agonist for acute pain treatment.

Example 1

An opioid-tolerant patient normally taking 150 mg of sustained release morphine twice a day was admitted requiring an emergency laparotomy and will be nil by mouth after surgery.

To prevent withdrawal, the usual oral 24 h opioid dose needs to be maintained, which is 300 mg of morphine. As the patient will be nil by mouth, this needs to be converted to an intravenous dose.

The conversion ratio for oral to intravenous morphine is between 3:1 and 2:1.

Using a 3:1 conversion ratio, the total intravenous dose over 24 h should be 100 mg, which is equivalent to a background infusion of 4 mg h^{-1}.

The PCA bolus dose can be started at 50% of the hourly dose of the background infusion, that is a bolus dose of 2 mg morphine with a lockout period of 5 min.

---

ii) Additional opioid for acute pain. For minor procedures, immediate release oral opioids, for example Oramorph and OxyNorm, can be used. The traditional approach is to administer a dose 1/6 of the patient's total 24 h usual opioid dose, given as required (PRN) up to 4-hourly. However, studies have shown that there is little or no relationship between the dose of immediate release opioid required to relieve breakthrough pain and the degree of opioid tolerance, with patients requiring smaller doses of immediate release opioid than would be expected from the traditionally calculated PRN dose. It is important to emphasise that the initial dose of PRN immediate-release opioid prescribed for breakthrough pain is just the starting point. These patients will need to be reviewed and the dose adjusted. The use of intravenous PCA is widely recommended for administering additional opioids for acute pain management as it allows individual dose titration and decreases workload for staff. Often patients will require increased bolus doses and possibly background infusions if they are unable to take their usual oral opioids. It can be difficult to know the optimal starting dose. One method is to base the size of the bolus on the patient's normal 24-h opioid requirement (see Example 1 above).

The opioid doses used in the examples are suggestions only and may not be suitable for all patients in all situations. Opioid-tolerant patients require more frequent assessments on the ward and it is likely that the initial PCA bolus dose or medication prescription chart may need to be altered depending on the patient's response, with doses possibly needing to be increased or decreased.

iii) Opioid rotation. This is where a patient is changed from one opioid to another, and is often used in the treatment of both chronic, non-cancer pain and cancer pain when patients develop intolerable opioid side effects or inadequate analgesia. Patients can develop tolerance to the analgesic effect of the initial opioid and in order to obtain sufficient analgesia, a greater dose of the original opioid is needed. However, we know that patients gain tolerance to both the beneficial effects of opioids, for example analgesia, and also to side effects, for example constipation and sedation, but the rate at which tolerance develops is not uniform. So, if a patient develops tolerance to the analgesic effect of the opioid at a greater rate than they develop tolerance to opioid side effects, they are often unable to tolerate the increased dose needed for analgesia due to excessive side effects. In this situation, changing to a different opioid can reduce side effects while resulting in an improvement in pain relief. The concept is based on the rationale that different opioids do not act to the same degree on the various opioid receptors; they are often metabolised differently and there is incomplete cross-tolerance between different types of opioids. The traditional approach is to calculate the dose of the new opioid by using opioid equi-analgesic dose conversion tables, and then reduce this dose by 30–50% because there is incomplete cross-tolerance among the different opioids. A number of published reviews have detailed the shortcomings of these tables and the studies used to derive them [3]. These studies used opioid-naïve subjects with single dose or limited dose ranges, and the study subjects had no concurrent illness or organ dysfunction. Therefore caution must be exercised when using these tables and, at best, they provide a rough guide. There is also evidence suggesting that the conventional practice of opioid rotation based on equi-analgesic tables may be an important factor in opioid-related deaths, particularly in chronic non-cancer pain patients. On the strength of this, a different approach to opioid rotation has been recommended for these patients. The current opioid is reduced by 10–30% and the new opioid introduced at the dose used for an opioid-naïve patient. There is gradual titration down of the longstanding opioid by 10–20% per week, and a gradual increase in the new opioid by 10–20% per week with the rotation occurring gradually over 4–8 weeks. This gradual opioid rotation can work well in primary care or in the outpatient setting of a chronic pain clinic but may not be particularly useful in the acute pain setting where a quicker rotation is needed.

3. Multidisciplinary team approach

Having a collaborative approach with other hospital specialities, such as drug and alcohol addiction services, palliative care and psychology, improves the quality of pain management in the opioid-tolerant patient. Regular review by the different specialities provides a more holistic service and may help to identify and deliver the patient's pain management requirements throughout their in-patient stay. Close liaison with the patient's general practitioner is also necessary to continue their pain management in the community setting.

4. Step-down analgesia plan

It is important to have a plan on how to convert the patient back from intravenous to oral opioids. One method is to calculate the patient's last 24-h consumption of intravenous opioids and convert this back to oral equivalents, then give 50% of this dose in a sustained-release oral preparation and have immediate release opioids prescribed on a PRN basis (Example 2). The dose of the immediate release opioids should be started at a maximum dose of 1/6 of the calculated total 24-h oral opioid equivalent. It is also important that the patient's general practitioner is made aware of the doses of opioids on discharge home and how these should be tapered down.

Example 2

A patient recovering from major surgery is now able to eat and drink, and the plan is to convert him from intravenous PCA morphine to oral morphine. He has used 60 mg of intravenous morphine in the last 24 h.

The conversion ratio of intravenous to oral morphine is 1:2 or 1:3.

60 mg of intravenous morphine is therefore equivalent to between 120 and 180 mg of oral morphine in a 24-h period. 50% of the calculated oral equivalent dose is given in a sustained release form, for example 30–45 mg of morphine sulphate sustained release, twice daily.

1/6 of the calculated oral equivalent dose is given in the immediate release form on a PRN basis, for example Oramorph 20–30 mg up to 4-hourly.

Management of patients on high-dose sublingual buprenorphine

High-dose sublingual buprenorphine is being increasingly used as a maintenance therapy in opioid addiction, as it is perceived to have fewer adverse effects and less social stigma. It is typically used in doses ranging from 8–32 mg every 2–3 days. Buprenorphine is a partial opioid agonist and its maximum effect at the μ-opioid receptor is less than that of a full agonist, producing a ceiling effect for respiratory depression and analgesia. It also has a very high opioid receptor affinity and its binding is not easily reversed by other opioids. These pharmacological properties make it an ideal drug for maintenance therapy for opioid addiction but can make the treatment of acute pain by conventional opioids difficult.

There is conflicting advice in the literature over whether to continue with the current dose of sublingual buprenorphine or to discontinue it and rotate to a conventional opioid such as methadone before surgery [4]. The current recommendations are to continue with the normal dose of sublingual buprenorphine, maximise the use of opioid-sparing adjuncts and use conventional opioid agonists to treat the acute pain. The doses of additional opioid analgesia may well be significantly higher than one would expect. In view of this, monitoring these patients in a high-dependency environment is advisable.

References

1. Breivik H, Collett B, Ventafridda V, Cohen R, Gallacher D. Survey of chronic pain in Europe: prevalence, impact on daily life and treatment. *European Journal of Pain* 2006; **10**: 287–333.
2. Loftus RW, Yeager MP, Clark JA, et al. Intra-operative ketamine reduces peri-operative opiate consumption in opiate-dependent patients with chronic back pain undergoing back surgery. *Anesthesiology* 2010; **113**: 639–646.
3. Natusch D. Equianalgesic doses of opioids – their use in clinical practice. *British Journal of Pain* 2012; **6**: 43–46.
4. Huxtable CA, Roberts LJ, Somogyi AA, Macintyre PE. Acute pain management of opioid-tolerant patients: a growing challenge. *Anaesthesia & Intensive Care* 2011; **39**: 804–823.

Further reading

Chapter 11.7: The opioid tolerant patient. In *ANZCA Acute Pain Management: Scientific Evidence*, 3rd edn. Melbourne: ANZCA & FPM, 2010. 422–427. http://www.fpm.anzca.edu.au/resources/books-and-publications/publications-1/Acute Pain - final version.pdf (accessed 21/4/2015).

Chapter 11.8: The patient with an addiction disorder. In *ANZCA Acute Pain Management: Scientific Evidence*, 3rd edn. Melbourne: ANZCA & FPM, 2010. 427–433. http://www.fpm.anzca.edu.au/resources/books-and-publications/publications-1/Acute Pain - final version.pdf (accessed 21/4/2015).

Mehta V, Langford RM, Acute pain management of opioid-dependent patients. *Anaesthesia* 2006; **61**: 269–276.

Roberts DM, Meyer-Witting M. High dose buprenorphine: perioperative precautions and management strategies. *Anaesthesia & Intensive Care* 2005; **33**: 17–25.

Roberts L. The opioid tolerant patient, including those with a substance abuse disorder. In Macintyre PE, Walker SM and Rowbotham DJ, eds. *Clinical Pain Management: Acute Pain*, 2nd edn. London: Hodder Arnold, 2008. 539–556.

Vigneault L, Turgeon AF, Côté D, et al. Perioperative intravenous lidocaine infusion for postoperative pain control: a meta-analysis of randomized controlled trials. *Canadian Journal of Anaesthesia* 2011; **58**: 22–37.

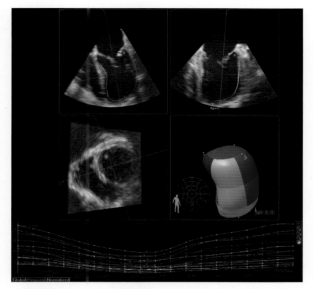

Figure 4.2 A multiplanar reconstruction of the left ventricle from a three-dimensional full-volume dataset. Semi-automated tracing of the left ventricle produces a surface rendered model, the 'jumping jellybean'. Graphic changes for each region of the 17-segment model of the left ventricle during the cardiac cycle are also shown. This patient had severe chronic mitral regurgitation. An end-diastolic volume of 205 mL and an end-systolic volume of 80 mL give a calculated stroke volume of 125 mL and an ejection fraction of 62%. Taken in isolation, these calculations overestimate cardiac performance, as they fail to take into account the mitral regurgitant fraction.

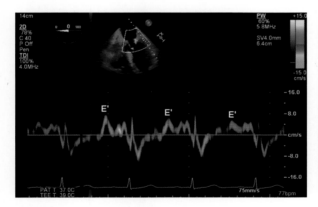

Figure 4.3 Tissue Doppler waveform obtained from the lateral mitral annulus. The peak early-diastolic mitral annular velocity (E′) is labelled. Combined with the peak early diastolic transmitral blood flow velocity (E, not shown), as the E/E′ ratio, it provides a reliable estimate of left ventricular filling pressure.

AAGBI Core Topics in Anaesthesia 2015, Edited by William Harrop-Griffiths, Richard Griffiths and Felicity Plaat.
© 2015 The Association of Anaesthetists of Great Britain and Ireland (AAGBI).
Published 2015 by John Wiley & Sons, Ltd.

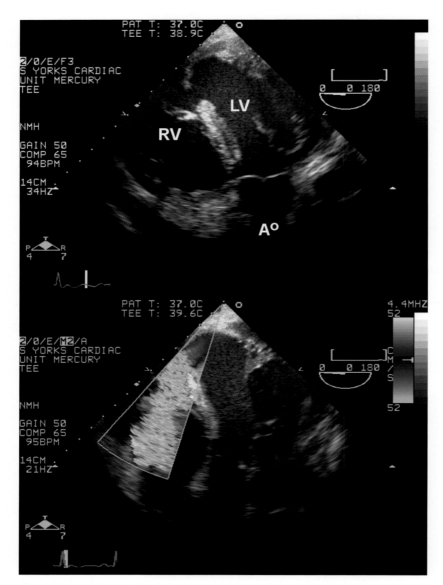

Figure 4.4 Transoesophageal, deep transgastric, long axis view obtained from a patient with a post-infarct ventriculoseptal defect. Top image: diastole with left (LV) and right (RV) ventricles. Bottom image: colour Doppler shows systolic blood flow across the defect.

CHAPTER 4

Echocardiography and Anaesthesia

Jonathan H. Rosser and Nicholas J. Morgan-Hughes
Northern General Hospital, Sheffield, UK

Key points

- Ultrasound is now an integral part of anaesthesia and intensive care practice.
- There is growing acceptance of the concept of focused, point-of-care echocardiography in which a non-specialist echocardiographer performs a limited examination.
- Echocardiography is an invaluable tool for assessing persistent unexplained hypotension.
- Modern echo machines are increasingly portable, affordable and have high specifications.
- Three-dimensional echocardiography has recently been introduced and is having a significant impact on clinical practice.
- Increasing numbers of training courses and accreditation processes aimed at non-cardiac anaesthetists and intensivists are available.

Echocardiography uses ultrasound to create real-time images of the heart, and Doppler to assess blood flow and tissue motion. Echocardiography is usually performed using the transthoracic or transoesophageal routes. The first textbook of echocardiography was published in 1972, heralding its acceptance into mainstream cardiology practice. Over the past 20 years, anaesthetists have incorporated transoesophageal echocardiography into peri-operative practice for patients undergoing cardiac surgery. This has aided the development of more complex procedures and has improved postoperative management in the cardiac intensive care unit. Most cardio-thoracic anaesthetists who are appointed to substantive posts in the UK are now expected to have trained in transoesophageal echocardiography. The UK accreditation process in transoesophageal echocardiography, which is a joint venture between the British Society of Echocardiography and the

AAGBI Core Topics in Anaesthesia 2015, Edited by William Harrop-Griffiths,
Richard Griffiths and Felicity Plaat.
© 2015 The Association of Anaesthetists of Great Britain and Ireland (AAGBI).
Published 2015 by John Wiley & Sons, Ltd.

Association of Cardiothoracic Anaesthetists, has been running for over a decade.

More recently, there has been growing interest in the use of peri-operative echocardiography in patients undergoing non-cardiac surgery, and also in the acute care setting. The increased availability of high-specification, affordable ultrasound equipment has been a necessary precursor. There is also increasing acceptance of the concept of focused point-of-care echocardiography in which a non-specialist echocardiographer performs a limited examination in order to exclude or detect major pathology and to assess haemodynamic parameters. There are a number of national level courses teaching this approach that are endorsed by UK specialist societies including the British Society of Echocardiography and the Intensive Care Society. The aim of this chapter is to examine some of these developments in the context of current anaesthetic practice.

Before surgery

Echocardiography by anaesthetists in the pre-assessment clinic is well described in the literature. However, it is even more useful in patients presenting for non-elective surgery who are often elderly and more likely to have undiagnosed cardiovascular pathology. They are also more likely to present out-of-hours when departmental echocardiography is unlikely to be available. Focused echocardiography in this setting has the potential to guide pre-operative optimisation as well as intra-operative and postoperative management.

Patients presenting with fractured neck of femur form a high-risk group. A recent study identified a 12% incidence of moderate to severe aortic stenosis in unselected fractured neck of femur patients. In England, the recently introduced 'Best Practice Tariff' for hip fracture patients introduced a financial penalty if there is a delay of >36 h from admission to surgery. The performance of echocardiography in hip fracture patients with undiagnosed heart murmurs is controversial given that it may delay operative fixation. The relevance of recognising severe aortic stenosis before surgery is twofold. First, it allows appropriate modification of the anaesthetic technique, possibly combined with use of an uncemented prosthesis to avoid cement implantation syndrome. Second, it ensures the timely diagnosis of a potentially life-limiting treatable disease. A focused echocardiogram performed by a trauma anaesthetist as part of their pre-operative assessment is a potential solution to the problem.

In aortic stenosis, echocardiography is used to assess the anatomy of the aortic valve, grade stenosis severity, and assess left ventricular function. A two-dimensional examination can identify leaflet thickening, mobility

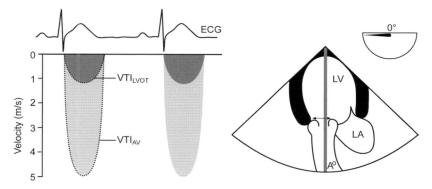

Figure 4.1 On the right is a two-dimensional echo image measuring the diameter of the left ventricular outflow tract (LVOT) (arrow). The cross-sectional area of the LVOT (CSA_{LVOT}) is assumed to be circular and is calculated from the diameter. The LVOT is also examined using Doppler (thick shaded line passing through open aortic valve). The resulting Doppler trace (left) shows a 'double envelope' signal. The higher velocity lighter envelope represents flow across the stenosed aortic valve and the lower velocity darker envelope represents flow through the LVOT. The peak velocity of blood through the stenosed valve is 5 m s^{-1}. Analysis software is used to trace around both velocity envelopes, allowing calculation of the velocity time integrals (VTIs) for the LVOT signal (VTI_{LVOT}) and the aortic signal (VTI_{AV}). Stroke volume is given by multiplying CSA_{LVOT} and VTI_{LVOT}. Given that flow through the outflow tract is the same as flow across the valve, the aortic valve area (AVA) can be calculated: $AVA = CSA_{LVOT} \times VTI_{LVOT}/VTI_{AV}$. *Source*: Brown and Morgan-Hughes, 2005 [*Continuing Education in Anaesthesia, Critical Care & Pain* 2005;5:1–4]. Reproduced with permission of Oxford University Press.

and evidence of calcification. An aortic valve with thin, mobile leaflets will not have significant stenosis. Doppler recordings are obtained from blood flow in the left ventricular outflow tract. The maximum velocity, which reflects flow across the valve at peak systole, can be used to assess severity, with a peak velocity >4 m s^{-1} representing severe stenosis. The drawback of using peak velocity for grading severity is that it is dependent on flow across the valve. Once the ventricle begins to fail secondary to the obstruction, severity will be underestimated. The most accurate method of assessing the degree of stenosis is by measuring the aortic valve area using the continuity equation (Figure 4.1). This is based on the principle that the stroke volume in the left ventricular outflow tract is equal to that passing through the stenotic valve. An aortic valve area <1 cm^2 represents severe stenosis. In patients with impaired left ventricular function, dobutamine stress echocardiography may be required to distinguish 'low-flow, low-gradient' aortic stenosis from mild aortic stenosis with coincidental left ventricular impairment.

The definition of what constitutes a focused echocardiogram varies, but most courses teaching focused echocardiography do not include the use of Doppler. A focused echocardiogram will therefore not offer a complete evaluation in a patient with aortic stenosis. Proponents of this approach argue that the important objective is not to anaesthetise a patient with aortic stenosis without being aware of the diagnosis. Once an initial diagnosis is made, appropriate precautions can be taken during fixation and precise quantification left to the cardiologists before possible valve replacement or transcatheter aortic valve implantation.

The burden of providing this service does not necessarily have to be carried by anaesthetists. Orthogeriatricians may be interested in acquiring the necessary skills. Alternatively, anaesthetic departments could employ a sonographer to service the trauma list and pre-assessment clinic while at the same time enhancing training opportunities for interested anaesthetists.

During surgery

The CardioQ™ oesophageal Doppler monitor can be thought of as a simple echo machine. A Doppler signal is recorded from the descending thoracic aorta using a small disposable probe, and a proprietary nomogram based on the patient's age, height and weight is used to calculate stroke volume. The Doppler signal is automatically traced, allowing continuous display of the stroke volume. This automation gives the CardioQ™ an advantage as a routine haemodynamic monitor over a conventional echo machine for which the software and probe design have historically been directed towards the manufacturer's primary market: diagnostic cardiology. Although stroke volume can be calculated using a conventional echo machine, obtaining repeated measurements is laborious. Another advantage of the CardioQ™ is that only minimal training is required before use. The CardioQ™ has been validated in terms of accuracy and can be coupled with a simple algorithm to guide goal-directed fluid administration.

The major advantage that echo has over conventional haemodynamic monitors is that as well as being able to provide a comprehensive haemodynamic snapshot, it provides a wealth of structural information, enabling diagnosis of the underlying cause of haemodynamic instability. The American Society of Anesthesiologists and the Society of Cardiovascular Anaesthesiologists published updated practice guidelines for peri-operative transoesophageal echocardiography in 2010. Based on a review of the literature (http://links.lww.com/ALN/A568) and on expert opinion, they recommended that for non-cardiac surgery, transoesophageal echocardiography could be used when the nature of the planned surgery or the patient's known or suspected cardiovascular pathology might result in severe haemodynamic, pulmonary or neurological compromise. Examples of the former are neurosurgical procedures in the semi-sitting position, liver transplantation, scoliosis surgery, endovascular aortic stent graft placement and resection of renal tumours that extend into the inferior vena cava. Examples of the latter might include patients with dynamic outflow tract obstruction secondary to hypertrophic cardiomyopathy and those with ventricular assist devices in place. They also recommend that if equipment and expertise are available, transoesophageal echocardiography should be used when unexplained, life-threatening intra-operative circulatory instability persists despite corrective therapy.

hTEE™ is a miniaturised, single-use, transoesophageal echo probe recently developed for haemodynamic monitoring in the peri-operative setting. It incorporates a monoplane transducer that can be used to generate three of the standard two-dimensional transoesophageal images of the heart.

The transgastric, mid-short axis view is a horizontal slice through the left ventricle at the level of the papillary muscles. This is the classic 'dancing doughnut' view and allows assessment of left ventricular wall motion and thickening. It can also be used to measure the left ventricular end-systolic and end-diastolic areas by planimetry. This in turn allows calculation of fractional area change as a surrogate for ventricular function. 'Eyeballing' of fractional area change by experienced operators accurately categorises systolic function and can be used as an alternative to formal measurement.

The second view displayed by the probe is the mid-oesophageal, four-chamber view. This is a coronal slice from the base to the apex of the heart and allows both atria and ventricles to be seen, and the motion of the interatrial septum to be assessed. Normally, the interatrial septum is bowed rightwards with a brief mid-systolic reversal. With increased left or right atrial pressure, the interatrial septum bulges to the opposite side throughout the cardiac cycle.

The third view is the mid-oesophageal, ascending aortic short axis view. This provides a transverse section through the superior vena cava. In mechanically ventilated patients, measurement of the maximum (expiratory) and minimum (inspiratory) superior vena caval diameter allows the collapsibility index to be calculated, which in turn identifies fluid responsiveness without the need for an initial fluid challenge.

By integrating the above information, it is possible to assess a patient's circulatory status rapidly (Table 4.1).

Fractional area change is load-dependent: severe mitral regurgitation will significantly offload the ventricle, thereby increasing fractional area change, and may lead to false assumptions about left ventricular function. Another issue is that the measurements do not take apical function into account. If an apical aneurysm were present but missed, the ventricle's systolic function would be overestimated.

Table 4.1 Typical echocardiographic profile of various haemodynamic states

	Possible pathology	Left ventricular contractility	LVEDA	LVESA	FAC	Other findings
Hypovolaemia	Dehydration, blood loss	↑	↓	↓	↑	'Kissing' papillary muscles
Vasoplegia	Sepsis	↑	↑	↓	←	
Acute left ventricular systolic dysfunction	Myocardial infarction, Takotsubo cardiomyopathy	↓	↑	←	↓	
Left ventricular diastolic dysfunction	Longstanding hypertension	↑	↓	↓	↑	IAS bowed to right
Acute cor pulmonale	Thrombo-embolism, venous air embolism	←	↓	↓	↓	IAS bowed to left, right heart dilated

LVEDA, left ventricular end diastolic area; LVESA, left ventricular end systolic area; FAC, fractional area change; IAS, interatrial septum.

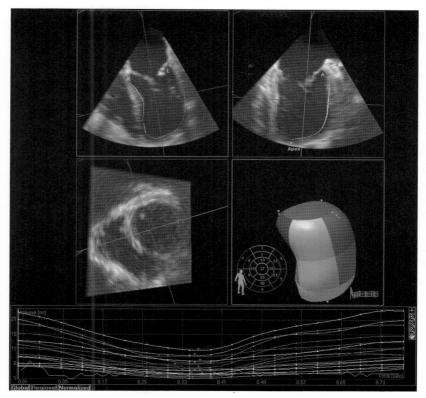

Figure 4.2 A multiplanar reconstruction of the left ventricle from a three-dimensional full-volume dataset. Semi-automated tracing of the left ventricle produces a surface rendered model, the 'jumping jellybean'. Graphic changes for each region of the 17-segment model of the left ventricle during the cardiac cycle are also shown. This patient had severe chronic mitral regurgitation. An end-diastolic volume of 205 mL and an end-systolic volume of 80 mL give a calculated stroke volume of 125 mL and an ejection fraction of 62%. Taken in isolation, these calculations overestimate cardiac performance, as they fail to take into account the mitral regurgitant fraction. (*For a colour version of this figure, see the colour plate section.*)

Conventional echo machines offer wider scope for assessment of the heart's function. Spectral Doppler can be used to assess stroke volume and valvular gradients. Three-dimensional echocardiography can image the entire left ventricle and can be used to provide accurate data on ventricular volumes and ejection fraction (Figure 4.2). Tissue Doppler imaging from the heart's base allows quantification of longitudinal cardiac motion and enables assessment of diastolic function and filling pressures (Figure 4.3).

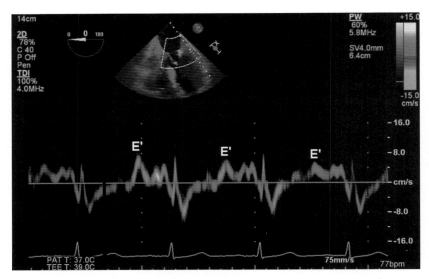

Figure 4.3 Tissue Doppler waveform obtained from the lateral mitral annulus. The peak early-diastolic mitral annular velocity (E′) is labelled. Combined with the peak early diastolic transmitral blood flow velocity (E, not shown), as the E/E′ ratio, it provides a reliable estimate of left ventricular filling pressure. (*For a colour version of this figure, see the colour plate section.*)

After surgery and in critical care

The American Society of Anesthesiologists and the Society of Cardiovascular Anesthesiologists practice guidelines for critical care recommend that transoesophageal echocardiography be used when diagnostic information that is expected to alter management cannot be obtained by transthoracic echocardiography or other modalities in a timely manner. General indications for critical care echocardiography are summarised in Table 4.2. The indications for urgent critical care echocardiography are persistent unexplained hypotension and persistent unexplained hypoxaemia. It is these two categories of patient that argue for echocardiography as a core skill for doctors working in critical care, as they require immediate assessment and action.

Persistent unexplained hypotension

Persistent unexplained hypotension has multiple causes. Its successful management depends upon accurate and rapid diagnosis, and this may not be possible with clinical examination alone. Echocardiography has been shown to be a safe and effective method of assessment in both the operating theatre and critical care environments. The use of echocardiography in assessing general causes of haemodynamic instability such as

Table 4.2 Possible indications for echocardiography in critical care patients

---

Adult respiratory distress syndrome
Thoracic trauma
Complications of myocardial infarction
Failure to wean from mechanical ventilation
Unexplained persistent haemodynamic instability*
Mechanical circulatory support
Identification of embolic source
Suspected infective endocarditis
Suspected thrombo-embolism
Unexplained persistent hypoxaemia*
Before cardioversion

---

*Urgent indication.

hypovolaemia or vasoplegia has already been described. We now turn to structural causes of hypotension for which echocardiography can provide an accurate anatomical diagnosis. Some of these conditions are relatively rare. However, collectively, patients with these underlying causes represent an important group of critical care patients.

Left ventricular systolic dysfunction

Left ventricular systolic dysfunction may be acute or chronic. Chronic dysfunction will produce a global decrease in function and ventricular dilatation in order to maintain stroke volume at the expense of the ejection fraction. Acute dysfunction is less well-tolerated because ventricular remodelling has not occurred. Myocardial ischaemia or infarction will lead to regional wall motion abnormalities without compensatory dilatation of the ventricle, which can be readily seen on echo. Takotsubo cardiomyopathy is an increasingly recognised acute cardiomyopathy. It can be triggered by emotional and physical stresses, including surgery. The presentation is of sudden onset heart failure associated with ECG changes suggestive of an anterior myocardial infarction. Coronary angiography is typically normal with systolic bulging of the left ventricular apex and a hypercontractile base seen on echocardiography. It is the hallmark bulging out of the apex of the heart with preserved function of the base that earned the syndrome its name 'takotsubo', or 'octopus pot' cardiomyopathy in Japan, where it was first described. With appropriate supportive measures, it carries a good prognosis with recovery of left ventricular function being the norm.

Right ventricular dysfunction

The right ventricle pumps blood through the low-pressure pulmonary vasculature. It has significantly less muscle mass and reserve than the left ventricle. Its main method of compensation is by dilation. Chronic right ventricular dysfunction may be seen in both volume and pressure overload. Volume overload results from left to right shunts and right-sided valvular regurgitation. Pressure overload is caused by right-sided stenotic lesions or pulmonary hypertension. Pulmonary thrombo-embolism is the most common cause of acute right ventricular dysfunction. In suspected acute pulmonary embolus, computed tomography pulmonary angiography is the gold standard for diagnosis. If the patient is hypotensive and computed tomography is unavailable or deemed too high risk, thrombolysis should be considered if there is unequivocal echocardiographic evidence of acute cor pulmonale – a dilated, poorly contracting right ventricle with an interatrial septum that is bowed to the left throughout the cardiac cycle. Echocardiography may also display thrombus in transit, and transoesophageal echocardiography may visualise thrombus in the main or right pulmonary artery.

Severe mitral regurgitation

Severe mitral regurgitation can cause hypotension and pulmonary oedema. Causes of acute, severe mitral regurgitation include endocarditis and papillary muscle rupture (vide infra) secondary to myocardial infarction. Myocardial infarction may also lead to ventricular septal rupture or a contained free-wall rupture. Defects can be easily visualised with two-dimensional echo and abnormal flow demonstrated with colour Doppler (Figure 4.4).

Dynamic left ventricular outflow obstruction

Obstruction of the left ventricular outflow tract can severely impair cardiac output. Septal hypertrophy, low systemic vascular resistance, relative hypovolaemia and increased contractility (due to endogenous or exogenous inotropes) can all lead to an increased velocity through the outflow tract. This decreases the pressure in the outflow tract, pulling the anterior mitral valve leaflet forward (systolic anterior motion), causing outflow tract obstruction. Systolic anterior motion of the anterior mitral valve leaflet is also seen in hypertrophic obstructive cardiomyopathy and following cardiac surgery. Although the clinical picture of deterioration following the introduction of beta-agonist therapy may suggest the diagnosis, confirmation requires echocardiography.

Cardiac tamponade and aortic dissection

Echocardiography is the diagnostic modality of choice in cardiac tamponade. Medical causes of tamponade include malignancy, uraemia and infection, and usually result in circumferential collections of fluid in the pericardial space. Echocardiography can be used both for diagnosis and to guide paracentesis. Tamponade may also be seen in aortic dissection.

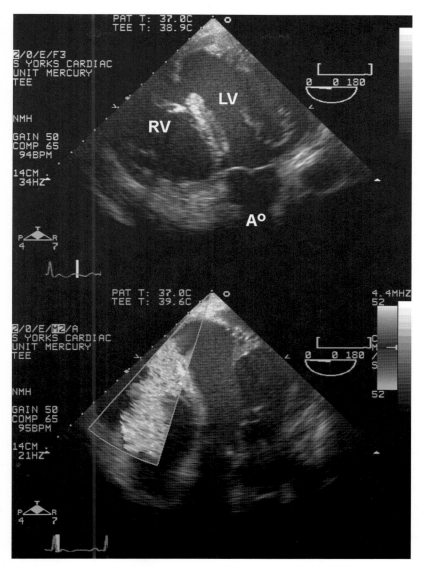

Figure 4.4 Transoesophageal, deep transgastric, long axis view obtained from a patient with a post-infarct ventriculoseptal defect. Top image: diastole with left (LV) and right (RV) ventricles. Bottom image: colour Doppler shows systolic blood flow across the defect. (*For a colour version of this figure, see the colour plate section.*)

Transoesophageal echocardiography is the technique of choice for diagnosis of aortic dissection. Most of the thoracic aorta can be visualised with transoesophageal echocardiography, and can display the location of the tear and the extent of the dissection, which have implications for both surgical and cardiopulmonary bypass techniques. Transthoracic echocardiography may be used to assess the proximal ascending aorta and for associated complications such as aortic regurgitation, regional wall motion abnormalities and cardiac tamponade.

Pleural effusion

Large pleural effusions can compress the heart and impair cardiac function. Pleural effusions can be easily visualised and quantified at echocardiography.

Illustrative clinical example

A 68-year-old man was admitted from home to the cardiac catheter suite for primary percutaneous coronary intervention. He had a 5-h history of chest pain and a 12-lead ECG showed ST segment elevation in the inferolateral leads. He suffered an asystolic cardiac arrest at the start of the procedure. Cardiac output was restored with an intravenous bolus of epinephrine (adrenaline) and temporary transvenous cardiac pacing. After cardiac arrest his oxygen saturations remained low, his trachea was intubated and his lungs ventilated. Coronary angiography showed total occlusion of a dominant right coronary artery. Coronary flow was restored, and a satisfactory angiographic result achieved after the deployment of three coronary stents. An intra-aortic balloon pump was inserted and he was transferred to the cardiac intensive care unit for further management. He required a F_iO_2 of 1.0 to maintain adequate oxygen saturations. Despite starting milrinone and norepinephrine (noradrenaline), he remained hypotensive with an invasive arterial blood pressure of 52/32 mmHg. In view of the persistent unexplained hypotension, a transoesophageal echocardiogram was performed. The first image obtained was a transgastric, mid-short axis view. This revealed hypermobility of the posteromedial papillary muscle, suggestive of papillary muscle rupture (Figure 4.5). The diagnosis was confirmed on subsequent views (Figure 4.6) and the presence of torrential mitral regurgitation demonstrated using colour Doppler of the mitral valve. The patient underwent an emergency mitral valve replacement. His postoperative course was complicated by ischaemic colitis and a sternal wound infection. He was discharged home 95 days after his initial admission.

Persistent unexplained hypoxaemia

Persistent unexplained hypoxaemia can result from the presence of a patent foramen ovale. A quarter of young adults have a patent foramen ovale. There is no deficiency of atrial septal tissue per se and, in the absence of left atrial dilation, the defect functions as a flap valve, only allowing right-to-left flow. Normally, left atrial pressure exceeds right atrial pressure and no shunting occurs. However, if right-sided pressures increase,

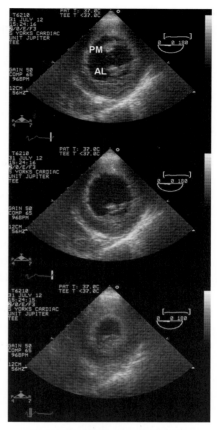

Figure 4.5 Transgastric, mid-short axis view obtained from a patient with a complete posteromedial papillary muscle rupture. Top image: end diastole with posteromedial (PM) and anterolateral (AL) papillary muscles. Middle image: phase of isovolumetric contraction with disappearance/hypermobility of the posteromedial papillary muscle suggestive of papillary muscle rupture. Lower image: end systole. Calculation of fractional area change in this patient would overestimate cardiac performance due to the presence of torrential mitral regurgitation.

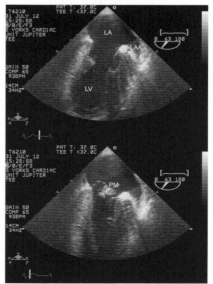

Figure 4.6 Long axis view obtained from the same patient as Figure 4.5. Top image: end diastole with left atrium (LA), left atrial appendage (LAA) and left ventricle (LV). Bottom image: end systole with the posteromedial papillary muscle (PM) seen prolapsing into the left atrium.

right-to-left shunting and therefore potential hypoxaemia can occur. Acutely, this may be seen with ventilator asynchrony or with high positive end-expiratory pressures in ventilated patients. It can also occur in adult respiratory distress patients with acute cor pulmonale or with right ventricular systolic dysfunction, particularly as part of the right ventricular infarction syndrome. The diagnosis should be considered in any intensive care patient in whom the degree of hypoxaemia appears disproportionate, and should be detectable by colour Doppler. Management might include a counterintuitive decrease in positive end-expiratory pressure and the re-establishment of spontaneous ventilation. If colour Doppler is inconclusive, bubble contrast administration can be helpful. Contrast is prepared by injecting 10 mL of a colloid solution back and forth between two Luer-lock syringes via a three-way tap before intravenous injection. There is no need to include air in either of the syringes. Theoretically, it is preferable to administer contrast via a lower limb vein as inferior vena caval blood is preferentially directed towards the atrial septum by the Eustachian valve, an embryological remnant of the fetal circulation. To establish the potential for right-to-left shunting, for instance before neurosurgery in the semi-sitting position, bubble contrast administration can be timed to coincide with the release of a Valsalva manoeuvre. The transient increase in right atrial pressure associated with cessation of a Valsalva manoeuvre opens the flap valve and bubble contrast can be seen passing into the left atrium.

Future trends

Manufacturers are increasingly tailoring machine design to the point-of-care environment with sealed control pads and automatic image optimisation. The use of ultrasound is now an integral part of anaesthesia and intensive care medical practice. The skill sets for ultrasound-guided regional anaesthesia, vascular access, lung ultrasound and focused echocardiography are not dissimilar, and once one technique has been learnt, the others quickly follow. In future it is likely that 'ultrasound-assisted examination' will be integrated into everyday clinical practice and given increased prominence in undergraduate and postgraduate medical training. Research is likely better to define clinical situations in which there are clear benefits from point-of-care echocardiography.

Further reading

British Society of Echocardiography. EchoCalc. (iPhone application). Version 2.0., 2014.
Intensive Care Society. Focused Intensive Care Echocardiography (FICE) Accreditation Pack. http://www.ics.ac.uk/EasysiteWeb/getresource.axd?AssetID=2057&type=full&servicetype=Attachment (accessed 12/5/2015).

Parnell A, Morgan-Hughes N, Russell C. ICE-BLU: the new e-LfH e-learning programme on echocardiography and basic lung ultrasound. *Bulletin of the Royal College of Anaesthetists* 2014; **87**: 44–45.

Royse CF, Canty DJ, Faris J, Haji DL, Veltman M, Royse A. Physician-performed ultrasound: the time has come for routine use in acute care medicine. *Anesthesia & Analgesia* 2012; **115**: 1007–1028.

Sidebotham D, Merry AF, Legget ME, Edwards ML. *Practical Perioperative Transesophageal Echocardiography With Critical Care Echocardiography*, 2nd edn. Philadelphia, PA: Elsevier, 2011.

USABCD A/S. FATE Card. (iPhone application). Version 1.2., 2012.

CHAPTER 5

Medico-Legal Aspects of Regional Anaesthesia

William T. Frame

Glasgow Royal Infirmary, Glasgow, UK

Key points

- Medical litigation is increasing at an alarming rate, with claims in England in 2010–2011 totalling 8655, with associated costs of £863 million. By 2012–2013, these figures had increased to 10,129 claims, with associated settlement costs of £1.309 billion.
- To be found guilty of medical negligence, it must be shown that the doctor adopted a course of action that no medical professional of ordinary skill would have taken if acting with ordinary care.
- The pre-operative visit is important in terms of striking a good rapport with the patient and in order to discuss the benefits and risks of the proposed anaesthetic technique. This is essential to meet the requirements of valid, informed consent.
- The standard of information required for valid consent has moved from the *reasonable doctor* standard to the *reasonable patient* standard.
- Chlorhexidine solutions are the most effective method of skin cleansing before regional anaesthesia. However, chlorhexidine is neurotoxic and contamination of block equipment must be avoided.
- All regional anaesthetic blocks should be performed with meticulous attention to detail. The optimum site of needle insertion should be carefully determined, and needles and catheters must be handled gently at all times.
- Block efficacy must be carefully checked before surgery commences.
- Surveillance is important in those patients who exhibit a neurological deficit in the postoperative period. Careful history taking, detailed clinical examination and, when indicated, magnetic resonance imaging are often sufficient to determine aetiology. Subsequent nerve conduction studies may be useful.

The use of regional anaesthesia, to include both central neuraxial and peripheral nerve blockade, either alone or in combination with general

---

AAGBI Core Topics in Anaesthesia 2015, Edited by William Harrop-Griffiths, Richard Griffiths and Felicity Plaat.
© 2015 The Association of Anaesthetists of Great Britain and Ireland (AAGBI).
Published 2015 by John Wiley & Sons, Ltd.

anaesthesia, has increased significantly over the last 10 years. There are several reasons to believe that this trend will continue, since regional anaesthesia has a good safety profile, provides excellent postoperative analgesia, a low incidence of postoperative nausea and vomiting and is an integral part of most enhanced recovery after surgery programmes. In addition, research is now focusing on the potential ability of the use of regional anaesthesia to have a beneficial impact on recurrence rates following surgery for certain types of malignant diseases such as cancer of the breast and prostate. If the promising results of these early studies are confirmed in the ongoing prospective multicentre trials, the use of regional anaesthesia will undoubtedly become even more widespread.

The incidence of litigation in all fields of medicine, including anaesthesia, is increasing at an alarming rate, with 10,129 claims of clinical negligence being reported in England between 2012 and 2013. This compares with 6652 claims during 2009–2010. Not surprisingly, the costs associated with these claims are also increasing, with the National Health Service Litigation Authority (NHSLA) paying out £787 million in 2009–2010, with the figure increasing to £1.309 billion in 2012–2013. The picture in Scotland is less bleak, with total costs of £35 million in 2009–2010, increasing to £60 million in 2012–2013. As the use of regional anaesthesia has become more widespread, the cost of litigation associated with this area of anaesthetic practice has also increased.

In order to prove that a doctor is guilty of medical negligence under UK law, the following must be established:

1 That the doctor owed the patient a duty of care.
2 That there was a breach of that duty of care.
3 That harm or detriment resulted, with any harm or detriment being entirely or largely due to the breach of the duty of care.

The third requirement, that of causation, is often difficult to prove, which can be fortunate for those practitioners whose patient management may have been found to have fallen below acceptable standards. The test case for medical negligence in England is Bolam versus Friern Hospital Management Committee (1957) with the equivalent in Scotland being Hunter versus Hanley (1955). Although the two cases are different in some respects, the legal test for both is very similar: in basic terms, to be proved guilty of medical negligence, it must be shown that the doctor adopted a course that no medical professional of ordinary skill would have taken if acting with ordinary care.

Szypula et al. have published information from the NHSLA's database about claims related to regional anaesthesia in England between 1995 and 2007 [1]. Although the dataset has a number of significant limitations, including a relative lack of clinical detail and no patient demographics, it does highlight the overall size of the problem and offers a useful insight into those areas of regional anaesthetic practice (and the associated costs) which are subject to claims for medical negligence. However, it should be emphasised that the dataset does not include any adverse events that did not result in legal action. This may limit its value in attempting accurately to predict the chances of litigation in relation to specific regional anaesthetic procedures. However, despite these unavoidable shortcomings, the major findings are of considerable interest:

- Regional anaesthesia accounted for 366 claims (44%) from a total of 841 anaesthesia-related claims.
- The total cost of claims associated with regional anaesthesia was £12.7 million, with peripheral nerve blockade accounting for only £0.12 million.
- 10% of claims included an allegation of lack of consent.
- 51% of claims were related to obstetric anaesthesia.
- 82% of the non-obstetric claims were related to neuraxial block.

The details of the central neuraxial block (CNB) claims were as follows:
- 326 claims (89% of all regional anaesthesia claims) were related to neuraxial block.
- 264 (81%) neuraxial claims were related to epidurals.
- 54 (17%) neuraxial claims were related to spinals.
- There were 89 claims for nerve damage.
- There were 45 claims for inadequate block.
- Seven out of eight claims related to combined spinal-epidural procedures were for alleged nerve damage.
- Epidural haematoma accounted for eight claims.
- There were 11 claims for neuraxial infection: seven for epidural abscess, two for spinal abscess and two for meningitis.

In sharp contrast, there were only 10 claims related to peripheral nerve blocks (PNBs), with upper limb blocks accounting for six of these. Two claims were for alleged intravenous injection of local anaesthetic solution, two for pneumothorax, one for nerve damage and one for infection from an indwelling catheter. All four lower limb block claims were for neurological damage.

The following discussion will highlight common pitfalls and strategies related to claims for medical negligence in relation to regional anaesthesia.

The pre-operative visit and consent

In a significant number of claims for medical negligence, poor communication following an adverse event is cited as a reason for the initiation of legal action. Pre-assessment clinics are now commonplace but the pre-operative visit remains the first opportunity that many patients have to meet the anaesthetist who will actually be providing their anaesthetic care. The anaesthetist must therefore use the pre-operative visit to establish a good rapport with the patient and to provide them with detailed information about the proposed anaesthetic. This conversation forms the basis of valid consent.

The requirements of valid consent are described by a number of sources, including the Association of Anaesthetists of Great Britain & Ireland (AAGBI) [2] and the General Medical Council (GMC) [3]. In basic terms, valid consent depends on the patient having the capacity to make a decision regarding their treatment and being able to do so without coercion. Capacity in legal terms requires that a patient must be able to understand and retain treatment information that is given to them. They must be able to weigh up the potential benefits and risks of the proposed treatment and to reach a decision about whether to give or withhold their consent. This decision does not have to stand up to logical analysis and it is immaterial whether the clinician agrees with it. In certain circumstances, valid consent may be obtained from patients who have not reached the age of 16 years, under the terms of 'Gillick' competence, if it is believed that they possess 'sufficient understanding and intelligence' to reach a decision regarding their treatment. With the introduction of the Adults with Incapacity (Scotland) Act 2000 and the Mental Capacity Act 2005, patients who lack capacity may now be given treatment so long as it can be shown that the proposed treatment is both necessary and in their best interests, in a wider sense than just medical best interests. This decision may be taken by the responsible clinician, by the courts or by an individual who has an appropriately registered power of attorney.

The standard of information necessary to meet the requirements of valid consent has changed significantly over the last 15–20 years. Previously, the information should have been that which a reasonable practitioner would provide as dictated by Bolam. The law now dictates that the 'reasonable patient' standard should be employed. The trend towards this standard was first seen in Australia in the case of Rogers versus Whitaker in 1992, in which the term 'material risk' was first used. A material risk is defined as:

- a risk to which a reasonable person in the patient's position, if warned of that risk, would be likely to attach significance, or
- a risk to which the medical practitioner is, or should reasonably be, aware that the particular patient, if warned of that risk, would be likely to attach significance.

A similar judgement followed in the UK six years later. In the case of Pearce versus United Bristol Healthcare NHS Trust (1998), the claimant suffered a stillbirth following a decision not to induce labour in an over-term pregnancy. She was not informed that non-intervention carried a small risk of stillbirth and the judgement in this case did, in effect, redefine the duty of disclosure to encompass those risks that a reasonable person, in the patient's position, would wish to know. More recently, in the case of Chester versus Afshar (2004), when a complication that had not been discussed occurred, the claim was upheld even though the claimant admitted she would have gone ahead with the procedure had she been told of the possibility of the complication occurring. This case, above all others, emphasises the importance of obtaining valid consent and ensuring that adequate documentation of the discussion with the patient regarding the risks and benefits of the proposed anaesthetic technique appears in either the anaesthetic record or in the patient's notes.

Although the legal requirements for consent have undergone many changes, the most important question remains unanswered. What should we tell our patients? Every patient is different but there is consensus that common complications must be discussed as well as rare but potentially serious ones. The latter might include those to which a particular patient would attach significance, for example, radial nerve damage in a piano player. In terms of regional anaesthesia, the discussion about risk should include mention of failure or inadequate block, local anaesthetic toxicity, infection and nerve injury. In addition, in the case of CNB, hypotension, headache and motor block should be mentioned. The pre-operative discussion should end with an invitation to the patient to ask questions and to raise any issues that may be of concern to them and which have not been covered. Finally, it should be remembered that the GMC's guidance [3] on patients who make it clear that they do not wish to receive a treatment such as regional anaesthesia is that these wishes and decisions should be clearly documented in the medical records.

Preparation for the performance of regional anaesthesia

On arrival in the operating theatre, the patient should have their identity, consent and the nature of the proposed surgery carefully checked in accordance with the Sign In step of the World Health Organization's Surgical Safety Checklist. As for all practical procedures, it is mandatory to prepare and check all equipment and drugs before embarking on any regional technique. In the case of CNBs and PNBs in which an indwelling catheter is to be inserted, a full aseptic technique, including the use of hat, facemask, gown and gloves, must be employed. For single shot PNBs, cleansing of the skin with antiseptic solution and the use of sterile gloves is acceptable.

Infection following CNB is rare. Only 15 epidural abscesses and three cases of bacterial meningitis were reported to the Royal College of

Anaesthetists' Third National Audit Project (NAP3) [4] in over 700,000 CNBs performed in the UK. However, poor aseptic technique was thought to be a factor in a number of these cases, and it should be remembered that an epidural abscess can lead to catastrophic consequences for the patient.

Skin cleansing can be achieved with either chlorhexidine-containing solutions or povidone-iodine. Chlorhexidine has been shown to be the more efficacious solution. Chlorhexidine 0.5% in 70% alcohol has a faster onset and longer duration of action than povidone-iodine, it retains its effectiveness even when blood contaminates the site of needle insertion, and adverse skin reactions are less common than with povidone-iodine. It should be emphasised that, in order to provide the maximum antiseptic action, chlorhexidine solution should be left to dry for at least 2 min before needle insertion. Hence skin cleansing should take place before preparation of drugs and equipment. This also reduces the risk of contamination of equipment by chlorhexidine.

Chlorhexidine is known to be neurotoxic in animal studies and it has also been implicated as the causative agent in cases involving permanent neurological deficit following CNB. In the first case, from the UK, the judge concluded that, on the balance of probability (although there appeared to be no hard evidence), the local anaesthetic solution that was injected into the subarachnoid space had been contaminated with chlorhexidine solution. In the second case, from Australia, 8 mL of colourless chlorhexidine solution was injected into the epidural space instead of normal saline, the colourless solution having been drawn up from a gallipot on the equipment tray. In both cases, the patients were left paraplegic.

These catastrophic cases emphasise two important points. First, it is mandatory that the anaesthetist's gloves, needles or any other equipment do not become contaminated with chlorhexidine during preparation for a regional technique, particularly a CNB. If a solution of chlorhexidine is used, the container should be placed as far away as possible from the rest of the equipment to avoid contamination. Should gloves or any equipment become contaminated, they must be disposed of and replacements obtained. Alternatively, chlorhexidine 0.5% spray can be used, as this minimises the potential contamination of equipment, assuming, of course, that the spray is allowed to dry before embarking on needle insertion. Second, in view of the sequence of events in Australia, it is sensible to avoid colourless chlorhexidine solutions. Coloured solutions are less likely to be mistaken for local anaesthetic or saline, and the addition of colour also helps ensure that no areas of skin are missed during cleansing with antiseptic solution. The AAGBI has produced guidance on this topic in which it recommends the use of chlorhexidine 0.5% rather than 2% for skin cleansing before regional anaesthesia [5].

Performance of a regional block

A major concern for patients undergoing surgery under regional anaesthesia, whether CNB or PNB, is that they will suffer neurological damage. When regional anaesthesia is used an added concern is that they will experience pain during surgery. It has been said that the recipe for successful regional anaesthesia is the right dose of the right drug in the right place. Sadly life is rarely that easy and a successful regional anaesthetic technique requires meticulous attention to detail, both in the performance of the block itself and in assessing its efficacy before allowing surgery to commence.

Central neuraxial blockade

NAP3 [4] quotes both 'optimistic' and 'pessimistic' figures for permanent harm following CNB. The pessimistic incidence of permanent harm following peri-operative epidural insertion is 1:5,800 and the optimistic figure being 1:12,000. The corresponding figures for spinal anaesthesia are 1:38,000 and 1:63,000.

Neurological deficit following CNB is usually due to trauma by the needle or epidural catheter, although a few cases involve compressive lesions, i.e. epidural abscess or haematoma. In the latter group, the prognosis is particularly poor even with early diagnosis of a space-occupying lesion.

Since the spinal cord in the average adult terminates at the level of the second lumbar vertebra, an interspace below the level of L2 is usually chosen for spinal needle insertion. Anaesthetists' estimations of the level of spinal needle insertion have been shown to be wildly inaccurate. In one study the spaces as identified by ultrasound were up to three interspaces higher than the anaesthetists' estimation [6]. Cases of damage to the conus medullaris associated with spinal anaesthesia have been reported [7]. It therefore makes sense to insert the spinal needle in as low an interspace as is practical, and definitely no higher than L3/4, a level that is taken to equate to Tuffier's line. Location of the midline is more challenging in the obese patient. If paraesthesia is elicited, this indicates that the needle tip has made contact with a spinal nerve root and hence is not in the midline. The entry of the needle into the subarachnoid space is thought to produce a small pressure wave that passes through the cerebrospinal fluid and causes the spinal cord and nerve roots to be pushed away from the point of the advancing needle. However, if the needle tip is more lateral, the nerve roots become less mobile as they approach the bony confines of the intervertebral foramen, increasing the risk of needle impingement. The site of resulting paraesthesia will indicate if the needle tip is to the left or right of the midline. Transient paraesthesia suggests that the advancing spinal needle has brushed against a nerve root. It is not usually associated with neurological sequelae.

Persistent paraesthesia or dysaesthesia may indicate that the spinal needle has transfixed the nerve root. The needle should be immediately removed to avoid permanent neurological deficit, although a temporary loss of function may result.

Transient paraesthesia, which returns upon injection of the local anaesthetic solution, indicates that the needle tip may be sited within the structure of the nerve root. The injection must be terminated immediately and the needle removed. Failure to do so may result in permanent neurological damage since injection of local anaesthetic solution into the nerve can disrupt its anatomical structure.

The efficacy of all CNBs must be carefully evaluated before the start of surgery. There has been considerable discussion over the years as to the optimum method of testing that a CNB is fit for purpose. Sensory block may be tested with pinprick, cold or light touch. Motor and sympathetic block must be evaluated. The modalities tested, how and when they are tested and the extent of the block should be documented. When regional techniques are used as the sole form of anaesthesia, surgery must be halted and alternative forms of analgesia and anaesthesia offered if the patient complains of pain. If further epidural drugs are given, time should be allowed for them to take effect, and the block should be rechecked before surgery is allowed to restart. Meticulous documentation of both what is offered and what is done is crucial under these circumstances, as the patient is unlikely to remember anything except their pain and distress.

Peripheral nerve blockade

The increasing use of PNBs over the last 5–10 years has undoubtedly been aided by the more widespread use of ultrasound guidance. The proven benefits of ultrasound-guided regional anaesthesia include the use of smaller volumes of local anaesthetic solution and a faster onset of block through more accurate placement of local anaesthetic solutions. However, patient safety has not yet been shown to have improved, and it appears that the incidence of neurological injury is essentially unchanged despite the ability to visualise the nerves during injection of the local anaesthetic.

The incidence of permanent neurological damage is estimated at around 1 in 5000 after peripheral blocks [8] although, in prospective studies, transient neurological abnormalities have been detected in up to 15% of patients. The discrepancy is likely due to temporary mononeuropathies detected during detailed clinical examination. Most neurological deficits related to PNB recover spontaneously: 95% within 6 weeks and 99% by 1 year. Although the safety profile of PNBs is good, it should never be forgotten that their complications can have a fatal outcome [9].

Why has the use of ultrasound to improve location of either single nerves or a nerve plexus not led to improvements in patient safety? Peripheral nerve blockade without ultrasound guidance is already extremely safe when conducted by experienced practitioners. Furthermore, peri-operative neurological deficits may be caused by a number of mechanisms unaffected by the use of ultrasound, such as poor patient positioning, pneumatic tourniquets, surgical trauma and nerve compression due to tissue swelling or haematoma after surgery.

As with all anaesthetic interventions, detailed documentation is vital. The antiseptic solution used, type of needle, nerve localisation method(s), local anaesthetic solutions injected (with any additives), and any paraesthesia elicited should be noted. In addition, if there is the possibility of neurological deficit before surgery, for example, diabetic neuropathy, a detailed clinical examination should be undertaken and any pre-existing deficit carefully described. It should not be forgotten that 'sick nerves' appear to be more susceptible to damage.

Postoperative care

For patients who have suffered a neurological problem, for whatever reason, the postoperative visit is extremely important and, if managed correctly, may prevent the initiation of the complaints process or legal action. Once again, good communication, both with the patient and with surgical colleagues, is the key. Clinical evaluation of a nerve injury must be thorough and should include:

- A full history that should include details of any paraesthesia, the duration of the block and whether the patient noticed any abnormality when the block wore off or, alternatively, when any deficit was first noticed. Other important points include the nature of any neurological deficit (motor, sensory or both), whether the symptoms are worsening or improving, and the extent of their functional impact.
- A detailed clinical examination is mandatory. This allows both full evaluation at the time of the examination and also assists in determining progress or deterioration during future visits. The clinical findings should, in the majority of cases, allow the anaesthetist to decide whether the neurological deficit is confined to a single nerve or whether it is affecting a nerve plexus or the spinal cord and/or nerve roots.
- With the increasing use of PNBs for anaesthesia, it may be difficult to determine whether a nerve injury is related directly to the surgery or to the PNB. In cases in which resolution of the injury is slower than expected or where the aetiology is in doubt, nerve conduction studies and electromyography are invaluable. Although the details of these are beyond the scope of this chapter, a neurophysiologist may be able to pinpoint the site of the nerve defect accurately and hence its likely causation.

- In patients who present with a CNS deficit after epidural or spinal anaesthesia, magnetic resonance imaging is the diagnostic tool of choice. However, clinical evaluation alone will frequently provide the likely diagnosis in these cases. In the presence of 'red flags', such as bladder or bowel dysfunction, or deterioration in the neurological picture, magnetic resonance imaging scanning must be urgently undertaken to exclude a compressive lesion such as an epidural haematoma or abscess. Delay in diagnosis has resulted in permanent neurological deficit that might have been avoided with earlier imaging.

After initial assessment, it is important to review progress regularly during the recovery phase. In those cases that include a significant functional deficit, physiotherapy and occupational therapy may help, and the importance of psychological support for the patient and the family should not be forgotten. These supportive measures not only assist in regaining the maximum possible function but, in those cases that lead to legal action, the level of the settlement may reflect the overall standard of care. Anaesthetists should involve neurologists at an early stage in diagnosis and management if a significant nerve lesion is identified.

How to reduce the likelihood of being sued

Despite the increasingly litigious environment in which we practise medicine, the likelihood of an anaesthetist being faced with a medico-legal action during their career remains small. Furthermore, if a civil action is embarked upon, the chances of the case actually reaching court are only around 1–2%. A few simple steps can help reduce the risk of patient harm and minimise the possibility of litigation:

- Effective communication with patients and colleagues is essential.
- There must be comprehensive documentation of the benefits and risks that were discussed regarding the proposed anaesthetic technique to indicate valid consent. Although adult patients have 3 years in which to initiate legal action for alleged medical negligence, the 3-year rule does not apply to children, and hence in a case of alleged negligence in relation to birth injury, legal proceedings may not be initiated for 10–12 years after the incident. This makes accurate record keeping vital, as no practitioner can have a detailed recollection of events after such a time interval.
- Perform a thorough evaluation of the regional block before the start of surgery. If you have doubts, it may well be inadequate and, if there is doubt in your own mind, your anxiety will be transmitted to the patient, whose anxiety levels will also escalate. This makes block failure even more likely.

- Make every attempt to perform regular postoperative surveillance, which facilitates early detection of neurological abnormalities and, where indicated, timely intervention.
- Finally, if a problem does arise that may lead to a medicolegal action, contact your medical defence organisation without delay. Their expertise is invaluable.

References

1. Szypula K, Ashpole KJ, Bogod D, et al. Litigation related to regional anaesthesia: an analysis of claims against the NHS in England 1995–2007. *Anaesthesia* 2010; **65**: 443–452.
2. Association of Anaesthetists of Great Britain & Ireland. *Consent for Anaesthesia*, 2nd edn, 2006. http://www.aagbi.org/publications/guidelines/docs/consent06.pdf (accessed 29/12/2014).
3. General Medical Council. *Consent: patients and doctors making decisions together*. 2008. http://www.gmc-uk.org/static/documents/content/Consent_-_English_0914.pdf (accessed 29/12/2014).
4. The Royal College of Anaesthetists. The 3rd National Audit Project of the Royal College of Anaesthetists. *National Audit of Major Complications of Central Neuraxial Block in the United Kingdom*, 2009. http://www.rcoa.ac.uk/nap3 (accessed 29/12/2014).
5. AAGBI, OAA, RA-UK, APAGBI. Safety guideline: skin antisepsis for central neuraxial blockade. *Anaesthesia* 2014; **69**: 1279–1286.
6. Broadbent CR, Maxwell WB, Ferrie R, Wilson DJ, Gawne-Cain M, Russell R. Ability of anaesthetists to identify a marked lumbar interspace. *Anaesthesia* 2000; **55**: 1122–1126.
7. Reynolds F. Damage to the conus medullaris following spinal anaesthesia. *Anaesthesia* 2001; **56**: 238–247.
8. Auroy Y, Benhamou D, Bargues L, et al. Major complications of regional anesthesia in France. The SOS Regional Anesthesia Hotline Service. *Anesthesiology* 2002; **97**: 1274–1280.
9. Yanovski B, Gaitini L, Volodarski D, Ben-David B. Catastrophic complication of an interscalene catheter for continuous peripheral nerve block analgesia. *Anaesthesia* 2012; **67**: 1166–1169.

Further reading

Barrington MJ, Snyder GL. Neurologic complications of regional anesthesia. *Current Opinion in Anesthesiology* 2011; **24**: 554–560.

Dennehy L, White S. Consent, assent and the importance of risk stratification. *British Journal of Anaesthesia* 2012; **109**: 40–46.

CHAPTER 6

Peri-Operative Use of Beta-Blockers: Yes or No?

Nanda Gopal Mandal
Peterborough City Hospital, Peterborough, UK

Key points

- The use of peri-operative beta-blockers reduces mortality and morbidity especially in high-risk cardiovascular cases. However, it is extremely important to administer them with consideration for timing, dose and duration in order to achieve the desired therapeutic benefits.
- Of the various beta-blockers, the cardioselective ones appear to be preferable in the peri-operative setting.
- Adverse outcomes with the use of peri-operative beta-blockers are more commonly seen in low-risk cardiovascular surgical patients who are given beta-blockers without appropriate dose titration and monitoring.
- More research is needed to define the role of beta-blockers in different clinical settings and circumstances.

The administration of peri-operative beta-blockers has been of interest to clinicians for almost four decades. In early clinical trials, beta-blockers were found to protect patients, decrease the incidence of peri-operative cardiovascular complications and provide better long-term survival. However, subsequent studies have shown either no benefit or greater morbidity and mortality despite decreases in the incidence of cardiovascular complications. The American College of Cardiology/American Heart Association (ACC/AHA) and European Society of Cardiology (ESC) have developed guidelines on the use of peri-operative beta-blockers. These guidelines have been revised in light of changing evidence. The current guidelines focus on risk stratification and dose adjustment according to haemodynamic responses. In spite of greater knowledge and understanding of the peri-operative use of beta-blockers, there are still many unanswered questions about their correct use in different clinical settings.

AAGBI Core Topics in Anaesthesia 2015, Edited by William Harrop-Griffiths,
Richard Griffiths and Felicity Plaat.
© 2015 The Association of Anaesthetists of Great Britain and Ireland (AAGBI).
Published 2015 by John Wiley & Sons, Ltd.

Further research is needed to identify clearly the subset of patients who are most likely to benefit from or be harmed by the administration of beta-blockers. A better understanding of genetic variability in patient responses to beta-blockers, different treatment modalities with beta-blockers and distinctions between different beta-blockers will help clinicians use these agents more appropriately.

Peri-operative cardiovascular complications comprise the most significant risks to patients undergoing major, non-cardiac surgery. A large number of patients with known coronary artery disease (CAD) or patients who are at risk of CAD suffer from peri-operative myocardial infarction (MI), congestive cardiac failure (CCF) and arrhythmias, leading to increased mortality and morbidity. Adverse cardiac events contribute to >50% of peri-operative deaths. These events have a considerable impact on length of hospital stay and the cost of care. Therefore, it is important to develop and implement strategies to decrease the incidence of these complications and thus minimise mortality, morbidity and cost of care.

Beta-blockers are used extensively in an attempt to minimise cardiovascular complications after surgery, particularly in high-risk patients undergoing major, non-cardiac surgical procedures under general anaesthesia. This chapter is intended to focus on the issues around the peri-operative use of beta-blockers. It includes a brief discussion of the pathophysiology of peri-operative myocardial damage, theories of how beta-blockers may prevent myocardial damage, peri-operative cardiovascular risk stratification, evidence of the usefulness of peri-operative beta-blockade, limitations of our current knowledge on this issue, the latest guidelines on peri-operative beta-blockers and future prospects for the prevention of cardiovascular complications in non-cardiac surgical patients by using cardioselective beta-blockers.

Pathophysiology of peri-operative myocardial damage

The pathophysiology of peri-operative myocardial damage has been much debated. It is thought that peri-operative ischaemic events are provoked by physiological derangements involving inflammatory mediators, hormones, sympathetic tone and an imbalance between oxygen supply and demand, which all occur as a result of surgery and anaesthesia. Surgical trauma, pain, anaemia and hypothermia are associated with increased levels of stress hormones. Plasma catecholamine levels correlate well with postoperative cardiac troponin increases and with graft occlusion after vascular surgery. However, it remains unclear whether they cause or result from these vascular events. Intraplaque inflammation plays a pivotal role in plaque instability and spontaneous acute coronary syndromes. Myocardial damage due to plaque rupture, thrombosis and occlusion can be seen in almost 50% of at-risk patients. However, recent investigations suggest that it is myocardial oxygen supply–demand imbalance that predominates in significance in the early postoperative phase. Most peri-operative MIs are silent, non-Q-wave events that are seen during the first 48 h after surgery when physiological derangements are at their greatest.

Mechanisms of the myocardial protective effects of beta-blockers

The mechanisms by which beta-blockers decrease the incidence of peri-operative cardiac complications remain unclear. A decrease in sympathetic tone resulting in a decrease in heart rate (increased perfusion time) and contractility (decrease in oxygen demand) along with coronary plaque sta-bilisation and the anti-arrhythmic action of beta-blockers are thought to be the main mechanisms by which they decrease cardiovascular risk. Beta-blockers are known to limit free radical production, decrease matrix met-alloproteinase activity and have an immunoregulatory role via effects on cytokine production. Many intracellular signalling pathways are associated with beta-adrenergic receptors. Cardiac muscle toxicity and apoptosis (pro-grammed cell death) are mediated predominantly via beta-1 receptor acti-vation. Hence, blocking these receptors with beta-blockers may have an effect on the response to reperfusion cell injury and cellular death.

Risk assessment for peri-operative cardiovascular mortality and morbidity

A prospective study by Goldman et al. [1] of 1,001 patients aged >40 years found that the overall risk of postoperative cardiac complications or death was 5.8%. Although subsequent reviews produced different mortality and morbidity statistics, it became clear that patients with underlying cardio-vascular diseases have an increased risk of peri-operative cardiac compli-cations. About 61% of patients who suffer peri-operative MI or cardiac arrest die within 30 days of surgery [2]. Risk stratification for adverse peri-operative myocardial events should be an integral part of the assessment of any patient before surgery. An evaluation in the pre-operative period should support the development of a strategy to minimise peri-operative complications and provide an assurance of better long-term outcome. Rou-tinely, the identification of high-risk patients is conducted with history, physical examination and estimation of functional capacity. However, for an objective assessment, validated risk scores that are based on clinical information and laboratory tests are widely used.

Since Goldman et al. [1] first proposed a risk model, several cardiac risk indices have been published. The Revised Cardiac Risk Index (RCRI) proposed by Lee et al. [3] is a risk model that is widely used as an objective assessment tool. The RCRI was derived and validated with a cohort of 4,315 patients. Observations made on 2,893 patients undergoing elective major non-cardiac procedures allowed the identification of six independent predictors of major cardiac complications, which were then validated in a cohort of 1,422 patients. The RCRI provides better predictive value than the original Goldman index or Detsky modified risk index. To calculate RCRI, one point is assigned for each of the following six variables: high-risk surgery (intraperitoneal, intrathoracic or supra-inguinal vascular procedures); history of ischaemic heart disease; history of heart failure; history of cerebrovascular disease; diabetes mellitus requiring insulin and; serum creatinine >2 mg dL^{-1}. However, with advances in minimally invasive surgery it is uncertain how relevant the categorisation of surgery is in assessing risk using the RCRI. Patients with a RCRI of ≥ 3 are considered to be high-risk, and those with a RCRI of 1 or 2 fall into the intermediate risk group. Risk estimation based on RCRI has been tested and validated as an accurate estimation of risk. The risks of major cardiac events, including MI, pulmonary oedema, ventricular fibrillation, primary cardiac arrest and complete heart block, in the presence and absence of beta-blockade are shown in Table 6.1 [3].

More recently, the National Surgical Quality Improvement Programme (NSQIP) model has been found to be a reliable predictor for cardiac risk assessment [2]. The NSQIP is the largest prospective clinical national surgical database and the NSQIP model is based on the statistical analysis of a database that includes $>400,000$ patients. Parameters such as ASA physical status, dependent functional status, age, abnormal creatinine (>1.5 mg dL^{-1}) and type of surgery are associated with cardiac risk after surgery. The

Table 6.1 Risk stratification with or without beta-blockers

Risk group	Revised Cardiac Risk Index score*	Risk of major cardiac events without beta-blockers	Risk of major cardiac events with beta-blockers
Low risk	0	0.4–1.0%	<1%
Intermediate risk	1 to 2	2.2–6.6%	0.8–1.6%
High risk	≥3	>9%	>3%

*Range of possible scores: 0–6.

NSQIP model has a higher predictive accuracy (C-statistic of 0.874) than the RCRI (C-statistic of 0.747).

Use of peri-operative beta-blockers in non-cardiac surgery: evidence of efficacy and safety

Earlier studies demonstrated that beta-blocker withdrawal was associated with tachycardia and an increased incidence of myocardial ischaemia, which justified the continued use of beta-blockers during the peri-operative period [4]. Subsequently, there has been an evolution of the literature on the use of peri-operative beta-blockers. In a placebo-controlled study of 200 patients with CAD or with risk factors for CAD, pre-operative use of atenolol was found to be effective in decreasing overall mortality and the incidence of cardiovascular complications for 2 years after discharge [5]. Overall mortality was significantly lower in the atenolol group at all points of follow up: 6 months (0% vs 8%), 1 year (3% vs 14%), 2 years (10% vs 21%). There was no difference in short-term outcome. However, the study excluded those patients who died in the immediate postoperative period. If these patients had been included in the analysis, the difference in death rate would not have been statistically significant. This study was criticised on the grounds of inadequate randomisation, small sample size, lack of an intention to treat analysis and lack of an early clinical difference.

A multicentre, randomised, non-blinded, placebo-controlled trial (DECREASE) using bisoprolol found a decrease in peri-operative death or non-fatal MI at 30 days [6]. This study included 112 patients who were selected from a large cohort of 1,351 patients with high-risk clinical features and abnormal dobutamine echocardiography. The patients in this study had at least one clinical marker of cardiac risk: MI, diabetes, CCF, angina, aged >70 years or poor functional status. Patients with extensive regional wall motion abnormalities were excluded from this study. Bisoprolol was started at least 1 week before surgery, and the dose was titrated to keep the heart rate <60 beats min^{-1}. Bisoprolol was continued for 30 days after surgery. The combined incidence of cardiac events was 3.4% in the bisoprolol group and 34% in placebo group. Treatment with bisoprolol resulted in a threefold decrease in the incidence of MI and cardiac death in high-risk patients. That was an almost 90% relative risk reduction for the combined outcome of cardiac death and non-fatal MI. The study was stopped early because the bisoprolol group had a highly significant lower rate of non-fatal MI and cardiac death at 30 days. The compelling results of the DECREASE trial group made a strong case for the use of beta-blockers in high-risk surgical patients. As a result, it was recommended that beta-blocker treatment be started 1–2 weeks before surgery and be continued for at least 2 weeks after surgery with a goal of keeping heart rate <70 beats min^{-1} before surgery and <80 beats min^{-1} in the immediate post-operative period. There were many drawbacks with this study. This study was not blinded and was inadequately randomised, which allowed potential bias and reporting error. It was terminated early and only focused on a specific group of patients. The magnitude of the efficacy of beta-blockade in decreasing adverse cardiac events was unexpected and was not seen in other studies, casting doubt upon the validity of the results.

After the publication of these two studies and several others, there was widespread enthusiasm for the use of beta-blockers in high-risk surgical patients undergoing vascular and other non-cardiac surgery. Boersma et al. [7] re-evaluated the DECREASE trial and analysed the characteristics of all 1,351 patients who had originally been considered for enrolment. They identified seven clinical risk factors that predicted adverse cardiac events: angina, MI, CCF, stroke, diabetes, renal failure and age >70 years. As the total number of clinical risk factors increased, peri-operative cardiac event rates also increased. For the entire cohort, patients taking beta-blockers had a lower risk of cardiac complications than those not taking beta-blockers (0.8% vs 2.3%). More importantly, in those patients with at least three risk factors, beta-blocker therapy was very effective in decreasing the incidence of cardiac events in those with new wall motion abnormalities in one to four segments (2.8% vs 33%). Those with intermediate risk (defined as one or two risk factors) had a very low event rate provided they were on beta-blockers. The risk of MI or death in the intermediate group was 0.9% with beta-blockade compared to 3% in those without.

Subsequent studies focused on the benefits of peri-operative beta-blockers in high-risk patients undergoing non-cardiac surgery. However, some of these studies did not produce favourable results, casting doubt on the efficacy and safety of peri-operative beta-blockade. A lack of definite benefit was demonstrated in two randomised studies involving specific patient populations: the Diabetic Postoperative Mortality and Morbidity study (DIPOM) [8] and the Metoprolol after Vascular Surgery (MaVS) study [9].

A retrospective cohort study [10] of 663,635 patients evaluated the effect of peri-operative beta-blocker therapy on peri-operative mortality based on pre-operative risk assessment using the RCRI. All patients were undergoing major non-cardiac surgery. In those patients with a low RCRI (0–1), peri-operative beta-blocker therapy increased the risk of in-hospital death, but in-hospital mortality was decreased in those patients with a RCRI ≥ 2. However, this study was retrospective, used a primarily administrative database and included emergency procedures.

A meta-analysis [11] of 22 randomised controlled trials (RCTs) with a total of 2,437 patients was inconclusive about the benefit of peri-operative beta-blockers. There was no effect on total or cardiovascular mortality based on statistical analysis using 99% confidence intervals for each relative risk. When outcomes were assessed with the more commonly used 95% confidence intervals, beta-blockers decreased the incidence of cardiovascular death, non-fatal MI and non-fatal cardiac arrest after 30 days. This analysis also noted that the use of beta-blockers was associated with a greater incidence of bradycardia and hypotension.

Two randomised trials by Brady et al. [12] and Juul et al. [13] fuelled the controversy. They found no significant benefit of beta-blockers in low- or intermediate-risk patients. However, in these trials, beta-blockers were only given within 24 hours of surgery and continued for only a short time into the postoperative period.

A population-based, retrospective cohort analysis [14] with 37,151 patients compared the long-acting beta-blocker atenolol with the shorter-acting agent metoprolol for elective surgery. The patient group treated with atenolol had significantly fewer postoperative MIs and deaths when compared with the group treated with metoprolol. Atenolol provided a 13% risk reduction over metoprolol for MI or death after adjusting for age, sex, type of surgery and use of furosemide, calcium channel blockers, angiotensin-converting enzyme inhibitors and statins.

The importance of heart rate control was illustrated in an observational study [15] of 272 patients undergoing elective, major vascular surgery. A significant reduction in peri-operative myocardial ischaemia and troponin T release were noted in those patients who had tight heart rate control and those who were treated with higher doses of beta-blockers. In addition, long-term mortality rates were lower in patients with lower heart rates. A similar observation was made in the DECREASE-II study [16] of heart rate control and risks of cardiac death or MI. The DECREASE-II trial was a prospective study of 1,476 patients who were undergoing major vascular surgery. In this trial, heart rate control to <65 beats min^{-1} was associated with significant risk reduction (1.3% vs 5.2%). An earlier systemic review [17] of five RCTs concluded that peri-operative beta-blockers should be started as long as 30 days before surgery to allow for titration of the dose to a target heart rate, and should be continued at least throughout hospitalisation or longer if adequate medical follow-up can be organised. The most marked decreases in peri-operative morbidity and mortality were seen in the highest-risk patients.

The ACC/AHA recommendations were first published in 2006. These practice guidelines recommended as a Class I indication (benefit clearly outweighs the risk) the peri-operative administration of beta-blockers to those patients who are already taking beta-blockers, and to vascular surgical patients with a positive stress test. They also recommended considering peri-operative beta-blocker therapy for patients undergoing intermediate-risk to high-risk procedures if pre-operative risk assessment identified them as having intermediate to higher cardiac risk, and for patients undergoing vascular surgery who were at low cardiac risk.

A systemic review and meta-analysis of 25 RCTs evaluated the use of peri-operative beta-blockers in patients undergoing non-cardiac surgery [18]. In this review, beta-blockers had no significant effects on mortality, acute MI, supraventricular arrhythmias or length of hospital stay. However, patients treated with beta-blockers had less peri-operative myocardial ischaemia and higher incidences of bradycardia and hypotension. More notably, the Perioperative Ischemic Evaluation Trial (POISE) [19] was conducted to investigate the effects of peri-operative beta-blockade in patients with known atherosclerosis or with risks for atherosclerosis. This was a large-scale RCT of peri-operative beta-blockade in 8,351 patients. The inclusion criteria were patients with CAD who were not on beta-blockers, those who had peripheral vascular disease, stroke, CCF within 3 years, major vascular surgery or three or more of seven risk factors (intrathoracic or intraperitoneal surgery, transient ischaemic attack, CCF, diabetes mellitus, creatinine ≥ 2 mg dL^{-1}, age >70 years, emergency or urgent surgery) undergoing non-cardiac surgery. The patients were randomised to receive either extended-release metoprolol succinate or placebo 2–4 h before surgery and continued for 30 days after surgery. The primary endpoint of this trial was a composite of cardiovascular death, non-fatal MI and non-fatal cardiac arrest at 30 days. At follow-up 30 days after surgery, significantly fewer patients treated with metoprolol reached the primary end-point (5.8% vs 6.9%). However, a significantly higher incidence of bradycardia (6.6% vs 2.4%), hypotension (15% vs 9.7%), stroke (1.0% vs 0.5%) and total mortality (3.1% vs 2.3%) was seen in the metoprolol group. The major contributors to the higher mortality rate in the metoprolol group appeared to be stroke and sepsis. How beta-blockers increase the risk of sepsis remains unclear. Drug-induced hypotension might be a predisposing factor for developing infections, or perhaps beta-blockers may mask the tachycardia associated with infection and thereby delay diagnosis. Many argued that the unfavourable outcome was due to the beta-blocker dose and the dose titration regime, which were too high and too aggressive, especially for patients who had never taken beta-blockers before. Additionally, the medication was started only a few hours before surgery and hence dose adjustment according to the response was not an option.

The POISE study is the largest trial conducted to date that addresses the issue of peri-operative beta-blockade in patients undergoing non-cardiac surgery. This study used a relatively large dose of metoprolol started only a few hours before surgery. In many of the meta-analyses conducted since its publication, POISE data account for a significant majority of the patients. Meta-analyses of trials including data from the POISE study have confirmed similarities in results and consistency with POISE findings. These analyses confirm a risk reduction in non-fatal MI with beta-blockers, but an increased risk of death and non-fatal stroke.

The DECREASE-IV [20] trial was performed on 1066 intermediate-risk patients who were undergoing vascular surgery. They were treated with either bisoprolol and/or fluvastatin or double placebo. Patients with bisoprolol had a significantly lower incidence of 30-day cardiac death and non-fatal MI (2.1% vs 6.0%). No difference was noted between bisoprolol and placebo in the incidence of beta-blocker-related safety end points. There was a lack of blinding and the study was terminated early due to slow enrolment.

Limitations of the studies

The papers published to date lack sufficient power to provide a clear answer about the role of peri-operative beta-blockade. Although there is some evidence of their usefulness in high-risk patients, methodological limitations prevent definitive conclusions. The exact role of peri-operative beta-blockers in intermediate-risk or low-risk patients has not been identified. Although there is a number of beta-blockers in clinical use, no single agent, dose, timing, duration or route of administration has been shown to be the most effective. Most of the positive studies are based on bisoprolol or atenolol, and some of the negative studies used metoprolol. As different studies used different population sets and dosing regimens, it is difficult to recommend any particular drug.

A recent analysis in vascular surgical patients suggests that a composite cardiovascular benefit is seen if the beta-blockers are started at least 1 week before surgery [21]. However, it is still uncertain whether this finding remains valid for other population groups or for different beta-blockers.

Genetic variation influences clinical responses to beta-blocker therapy, as variations in the adrenergic signalling pathway are common. They have a major impact on adrenergic receptor function and the efficacy of beta-blockers. Genetic variations in the cytochrome P450 enzyme system, which is responsible for the metabolism of most beta-blockers, are significant. Variations in metabolism can lead to either poor metabolising of beta-blockers or their rapid degradation. The inconsistency of the results of clinical studies may be due in part to heterogeneous responses to beta-blockers.

Patients with chronic obstructive pulmonary disease or bronchial asthma can also suffer from cardiovascular disease. However, few are given peri-operative beta-blockers because of concern that these drugs will aggravate bronchospasm. There is anecdotal evidence that carefully selected patients from this group can tolerate cardioselective beta-blockers without experiencing respiratory complications. However, the range of peri-operative benefits of beta-blockade in these patients needs further investigation.

Table 6.2 American College of Cardiology and American Heart Association Guidelines (2009): summary of recommendations for peri-operative beta-blocker therapy [23]

Size of treatment effect	Indications for peri-operative beta-blockers
Class I (Benefit >> Risk) Class IIa (Benefit > Risk)	• Patients already receiving beta-blockers for angina, arrhythmia and hypertension • Patients with coronary artery disease undergoing vascular surgery • Patients with multiple clinical risk factors undergoing vascular surgery • Patients with coronary artery disease or multiple clinical risk factors undergoing intermediate to high-risk procedures

Current guidelines

There are two international guidelines that were published in 2009 following the POISE study. The ESC guideline, endorsed by the European Society of Anaesthesiology (ESA), was published in August 2009 [22]. This guideline addressed many issues relating to the management of patients with heart disease, especially coronary heart disease, presenting for non-cardiac surgery, and included a section on peri-operative beta-blockade. The second guideline [23] was published in November 2009 by the ACC/AHA and featured an update on peri-operative beta-blockers (Table 6.2). Both of these guidelines include definitions of the classification of recommendations and the accompanying level of evidence.

The ESC guideline recommends beta-blockers for patients undergoing high-risk surgery without reference to the severity of cardiac risk. The ACC/AHA recommends beta-blockers in high-risk patients undergoing vascular surgery and are more restrictive. For intermediate-risk surgery, both these guidelines provide information on the use of beta-blockers. The ACC/AHA guideline requires the presence of CAD or high cardiac risk. The ACC/AHA guideline also states that in the presence of a single clinical risk factor, the usefulness of beta-blockers is uncertain for patients undergoing intermediate-risk procedures or vascular surgery. The ESC guideline suggests that patients having low-risk surgery with risk factors should be considered for beta-blockers, but there is no such recommendation in the ACC/AHA guideline. The ACC/AHA guidelines added another Class III (Risk ≥ Benefit) recommendation as follows: 'routine administration of high-dose beta-blockers in the absence of dose titration is not useful and may be harmful to patients not currently taking beta-blockers who are undergoing non-cardiac surgery'.

A recent systematic review [24] found that peri-operative beta-blockade started within a day prior to non-cardiac surgery reduces non-fatal MI. However, it can increase the risk of stroke, death, hypotension and bradycardia. This review concluded that in the absence of controversial studies (POISE and DECREASE), there is insufficient robust data on the efficacy and safety of peri-operative beta-blocker regimens that use agents aside from metoprolol or initiate treatment 2 to 45 days prior to surgery. Following the publication of this review, the USA guidelines were published by the ACC/AHA [25] on the use on peri-operative beta-blockers.

The main recommendations of these guidelines are:

1 Beta-blockers should be continued in patients undergoing surgery who have been on beta-blockers chronically.
2 It is reasonable for the management of beta-blockers after surgery to be guided by clinical circumstances, independent of when the agent was started.
3 In patients with intermediate-risk or high-risk for myocardial ischemia noted in pre-operative risk stratification tests, it may be reasonable to begin peri-operative beta-blockers.
4 In patients with three or more RCRI risk factors, e.g. diabetes mellitus, heart failure, CAD, renal insufficiency, cerebrovascular accident, it may be reasonable to begin beta-blockers before surgery.
5 In patients with a compelling long-term indication for beta-blocker therapy but no other RCRI risk factors, initiating beta-blockers in the peri-operative setting as an approach to reduce peri-operative risk is of uncertain benefit.
6 In patients in whom beta-blocker therapy is initiated, it may be reasonable to begin peri-operative beta-blockers long enough in advance to assess safety and tolerability, preferably more than 1 day before surgery.
7 Beta-blocker therapy should not be started on the day of surgery in patients who are not on beta-blockers, particularly at high initial doses, in long-acting form, and if there are no plans for dose titration or monitoring for adverse events.

In the 2014 European joint guidelines from ESC/ESA [26], beta-blockers are not recommended in patients without clinical risk factors because they may increase the risk of cardiovascular complications. In these European guidelines [26], controversial studies, e.g. DECREASE, were excluded in order to formulate new recommendations. However, the USA guidelines [25] included the DECREASE studies in its sensitivity analysis, but did not include the findings in the new practice guidelines.

Where do we go from here?

The results of published studies are inconsistent and sometimes confusing as a result of fundamental differences in study design. Only limited reliable conclusions can be drawn from the currently available data. The marked heterogeneity and insufficient power of the small number of randomised trials make comparisons difficult, if not inappropriate. Although there have been significant developments in our knowledge about the use of peri-operative beta-blockers, the optimal strategy in different clinical settings is still a matter of debate. The POISE trial has shown that acute administration of high-dose beta-blockers may be associated with increased mortality and morbidity, whereas the DECREASE study tells us that a low dose of a long-acting beta-blocker given by titration to produce effects at least 7 days before surgery can provide overall benefits in the peri-operative period.

The current data do not provide strong support for the routine use of peri-operative beta-blockers in low-risk or intermediate-risk patients who are undergoing non-cardiac surgery. It is certain that the use of peri-operative beta-blockers decreases the incidence of cardiovascular complications in high-risk patients (RCRI >2) or in patients with significant pre-operative myocardial ischaemia. This idea has been further reinforced from the findings of another recent study [27], in which early use of peri-operative beta-blockers was associated with significantly lower rates of 30-day mortality and cardiac morbidity in patients at elevated baseline cardiac risk undergoing non-vascular surgery. Hence, this group of patients should be given peri-operative beta-blockers, with possible continuation in the postoperative period.

Beta-blockers should be started early, at least 2 weeks (preferably 30 days) before the proposed surgical intervention in order to allow gradual titration of dosage to achieve a desired heart rate and degree of blood pressure control. The decrease in cardiovascular risk is greater when a long-acting beta-blocker (atenolol) is chosen rather than a short-acting one (metoprolol), and when the target heart rate is <65 beats min^{-1}.

The importance of maintaining peri-operative cardiovascular stability cannot be overemphasised. It is extremely important to control heart rate, arterial blood pressure and cardiac output in trying to balance increased left ventricular diastolic perfusion time from a low heart rate while maintaining adequate coronary perfusion pressure. All causes of tachycardia, hypertension, hypotension, anaemia and pain should be treated aggressively. In fact, intravenous beta-blockers have been used to control tachycardia, hypertension and ischaemia with results comparable to or better than those reported with prophylactic beta-blockers.

Patients already on beta-blockers before surgery should continue with their medication at least throughout the peri-operative period. A recent publication [28] reconfirmed that the continuation of beta-blockers on the day of and after surgery was associated with fewer cardiac events and a lower 90-day mortality. A focus on beta-blocker continuation and compliance with medication instructions during the peri-operative period is a worthwhile quality improvement target.

The allegations of use of fictitious data and scientific misconduct against Don Poldermans have left many clinicians in a state of limbo. Poldermans, one of the best-known researchers in peri-operative medicine, heavily influenced the clinical use of peri-operative beta-blockers in non-cardiac surgery. Two recent reviews [26,29] in which those controversial studies were excluded from the analysis, did not find any particular benefit of peri-operative beta-blocker usage. In fact one meta-analysis [29] with 11 credible RCTs indicated that peri-operative initiation of beta-blockers increased mortality by 27%. The controversy around the issue of peri-operative beta-blockers will continue and it is unlikely to be resolved soon. Meanwhile, careful attention to both patient risk and beta-blocker profile is important for safe and effective implementation of this therapy. Current research into the usefulness of alpha-2 adrenergic agonists, statins and antiplatelet agents with potential utility in the peri-operative setting will be another direction for cardiovascular risk optimisation. A few recommendations on this issue have recently been published [25, 26] and it is likely that more clearly defined recommendations are to come in the future.

Conclusions

The consequences of peri-operative cardiovascular complications are significant, and the number of patients at risk of these complications is going to increase year on year because of the ageing population. There is no proven benefit to peri-operative beta-blocker administration without prior risk stratification. The POISE trial shows that some patients can suffer from complications as a result of beta-blockade. However, certain risk groups may well benefit from the use of peri-operative beta-blockers. It is important to identify the appropriate target population. To achieve this, risk must be assessed, sound guidelines should be developed and timely preventative therapy with appropriate pharmacological agents should be instituted. The decision to give beta-blockers should be made on a case-by-case basis after appropriate risk stratification. Further research is needed to characterise the appropriate therapeutic regime and mode of administration to achieve the best outcomes.

References

1. Goldman L, Caldera DL, Nussbaum SR, et al. Multifactorial index of cardiac risk in noncardiac surgical procedures. *New England Journal of Medicine* 1977; **297**: 845–850.

2. Gupta PK, Gupta H, Sundaram A, et al. Development and validation of a risk calculator for prediction of cardiac risk after surgery. *Circulation* 2011; **124**: 381–387.

3. Lee TH, Marcantonio ER, Mangione CM, et al. Derivation and prospective validation of a simple index for prediction of cardiac risk of major noncardiac surgery. *Circulation* 1999; **100**: 1043–1049.

4. Prys-Roberts C, Meloche R, Foëx P. Studies of anaesthesia in relation to hypertension. I. Cardiovascular responses of treated and untreated patients. *British Journal of Anaesthesia* 1971; **43**: 122–137.

5. Mangano DT, Layug EL, Wallace A, Tateo I. Effect of atenolol on mortality and cardiovascular morbidity after noncardiac surgery. Multicenter study of perioperative ischemic research group. *New England Journal of Medicine* 1996; **335**: 1713–1720.

6. Poldermans D, Boersma E, Bax JJ, et al. The effect of bisoprolol on perioperative mortality and myocardial infarction in high-risk patients undergoing vascular surgery. Dutch echocardiographic cardiac risk evaluation applying stress echocardiography study group. *New England Journal of Medicine* 1999; **341**: 1789–1794.

7. Boersma E, Poldermans D, Bax JJ, et al. Predictors of cardiac events after major vascular surgery: role of clinical characteristics, dobutamine echocardiography, and beta-blocker therapy. *Journal of the American Medical Association* 2001; **285**: 1865–1873.

8. Juul AB, Wetterslev J, Kofoed-Enevoldsen A, et al. The Diabetic Postoperative Mortality and Morbidity (DIPOM) trial: rationale and design of a multicenter, randomized, placebo-controlled, clinical trial of metoprolol for patients with diabetes mellitus who are undergoing major noncardiac surgery. *American Heart Journal* 2004; **147**: 677–683.

9. Yang H, Raymer K, Butler R, Parlow J, Roberts R. The effects of perioperative beta-blockade: results of the Metoprolol after Vascular Surgery (MaVS) study, a randomized controlled trial. *American Heart Journal* 2006; **152**: 983–990.

10. Lindenauer PK, Pekow K, Wang K, Mamidi DK, Gutierrez B, Benjamin EM. Perioperative beta-blocker therapy and mortality after major noncardiac surgery. *New England Journal of Medicine* 2005; **353**: 349–61.

11. Devereaux PJ, Beattie WS, Choi PT, et al. How strong is the evidence for the use of perioperative beta blockers in non-cardiac surgery? Systematic review and meta-analysis of randomised controlled trials. *British Medical Journal* 2005; **331**: 313–321.

12. Brady AR, Gibbs JS, Greenhalgh RM, Powell JT, Sydes MR. POBBLE trial investigators. Perioperative beta-blockade (POBBLE) for patients undergoing infrarenal vascular surgery; results of a randomized double-blind controlled trial. *Journal of Vascular Surgery* 2005; **41**: 602–609.

13. Juul AB, Wetterslev J, Gluud C, et al. Effect of perioperative beta blockade in patients with diabetes undergoing major non-cardiac surgery: randomised placebo controlled blinded multicentre trial. *British Medical Journal* 2006; **332**: 1482.

14. Redelmeier D, Scales D, Kopp A. Beta blockers for elective surgery in elderly patients: population based, retrospective cohort study. *British Medical Journal* 2005; **331**: 932.

15. Feringa HH, Bax JJ, Boersma E, et al. High-dose beta-blockers and tight heart rate control reduce myocardial ischemia and troponin T release in vascular surgery patients. *Circulation* 2006; **114**(1 suppl.): I344–I349.

16. Poldermans D, Bax JJ, Schouten O, et al. Should major vascular surgery be delayed because of preoperative cardiac testing in intermediate-risk patients receiving beta-blocker therapy with tight heart rate control? *Journal of the American College of Cardiology* 2006; **48**: 964–969.

17. Auerbach AD, Goldman L. Beta-blockers and reduction of cardiac events in noncardiac surgery: scientific review. *Journal of the American Medical Association* 2002; **287**: 1435–1444.

18. Wiesbauer F, Schlager O, Domanovits H, et al. Perioperative beta-blockers for preventing surgery-related mortality and morbidity: a systemic review and meta-analysis. *Anesthesia & Analgesia* 2007; **104**: 27–41.

19. POISE Study Group, Devereaux PJ, Yang H, et al. Effects of extended-release metoprolol succinate in patients undergoing non-cardiac surgery (POISE Trial): a randomised controlled trial. *Lancet* 2008; **371**: 1839–1847.

20. Dunkelgrun M, Boersma E, Schouten O, et al. Bisoprolol and fluvastatin for the reduction of perioperative cardiac mortality and myocardial infarction in intermediate-risk patients undergoing noncardiovascular surgery: a randomized controlled trial (DECREASE-IV). *Annals of Surgery* 2009; **249**: 921–926.

21. Flu WJ, van Kuijk JP, Chonchol M, et al. Timing of pre-operative beta-blocker treatment in vascular surgery patients: influence on postoperative outcome. *Journal of the American College of Cardiology* 2010; **56**: 1922–1929.

22. The Task Force for Preoperative Cardiac Risk Assessment and Perioperative Cardiac Management in Non-cardiac Surgery of the European Society of Cardiology (ESC) and endorsed by the European Society of Anaesthesiology (ESA). Guidelines for preoperative cardiac risk assessment and perioperative cardiac management in non-cardiac surgery. *European Heart Journal* 2009; **30**: 2769–812.

23. Fleischmann KE, Beckman JA, Buller CE, et al. ACCF/AHA focused update on perioperative beta blockade. *Journal of the American College of Cardiology* 2009; **54**: 2102–2128.

24. Wijeysundera DN, Duncan D, Nkonde-Price C, et al. Perioperative beta blockade in noncardiac surgery: a systematic review for the 2014 ACC/AHA guideline on perioperative cardiovascular evaluation and management of patients undergoing noncardiac surgery a report of the American College of Cardiology/American Heart Association task force on practice guidelines. *Journal of the American College of Cardiology* 2014; **64**: 2406–2425.

25. Fleisher LA, Fleischmann KE, Auerbach AD, et al. ACC/AHA guideline on perioperative cardiovascular evaluation and management of patients undergoing noncardiac surgery a report of the American College of Cardiology/American Heart Association task force on practice guidelines. *Journal of the American College of Cardiology* 2014; **64**: e77–e137

26. Kristensen SD, Knuuti J, Saraste A, et al. ESC/ESA guidelines on non-cardiac surgery: cardiovascular assessment and management: the joint task force on non-cardiac surgery: cardiovascular assessment and management of the European Society of Cardiology (ESC) and the European Society of Anaesthesiology (ESA). *European Heart Journal* 2014; **35**: 2383–431.

27. London MJ, Hur K, Schwartz GG, Henderson WG. Association of perioperative β-blockade with mortality and cardiovascular morbidity following major noncardiac surgery. *Journal of the American Medical Association* 2013; **309**: 1704–1713.

28. Kwon S, Thompson R, Florence M, et al. β-blocker continuation after non-cardiac surgery. A report from the surgical care and outcomes assessment program. *Archives of Surgery* 2012; **147**: 467–473.

29. Bouri S, Shun-Shin M, Cole GD, Mayet J, Francis DP. Meta-analysis of secure randomised controlled trials of β-blockade to prevent perioperative death in noncardiac surgery. *Heart* 2014; **100**: 456–464.

CHAPTER 7

Transfusion Requirements and the Older Person

Alexa Mannings[1] and Iain Moppett[2]

[1] Sheffield Teaching Hospitals NHS Foundation Trust, Sheffield, UK
[2] University of Nottingham and Nottingham University Hospitals NHS Trust, Nottingham, UK

Key points

- Anaemia is common in the general elderly population, with increasing prevalence in surgical populations.
- Approximately one third of patients fall into each category of anaemia: nutrient deficient, anaemia of chronic inflammation, unexplained.
- Anaemia is associated with a variety of morbidities and increased mortality in community cohort studies of elderly people.
- Anaemia is independently and significantly associated with mortality and morbidity in the peri-operative period.
- Transfusion thresholds in the elderly have little strong evidence to support them.
- Restrictive strategies in the postoperative period appear safe, except where there is significant or active cardiac disease.
- Intra-operative transfusion per se can be demonstrated to be harmful.
- Intra-operative transfusion is of benefit in the severely anaemic, and the mildly anaemic who suffer moderate blood loss.

Anaemia in the elderly

Prevalence

The World Health Organization (WHO) defines anaemia as a haemoglobin level of <120 g L^{-1} for non-pregnant women, and <130 g L^{-1} for men aged >15 years. Using this definition, a UK community-based population study of over 65-year-olds identified a prevalence of 14% for men, and 11% for women [1]. This is somewhat greater than a German population-based study using the WHO criteria, which identified a prevalence of 4.3% in both

---

AAGBI Core Topics in Anaesthesia 2015, Edited by William Harrop-Griffiths, Richard Griffiths and Felicity Plaat.
© 2015 The Association of Anaesthetists of Great Britain and Ireland (AAGBI).
Published 2015 by John Wiley & Sons, Ltd.

men and women aged over 65 [2], but similar to the community-based American National Health and Nutrition Examination Survey (NHANES) cohort of over 65-year-olds, which found an overall prevalence of anaemia of about 10%. In those aged over 85 years, 26% of men and 20% of women were anaemic. Anaemia was generally mild, with only 1.6% of men and 2.8% of women presenting with haemoglobin levels <110 g L^{-1} [3].

There is considerable variance in the reported prevalence of anaemia, reflecting the heterogeneity of the populations observed. The very elderly, and those resident in nursing homes, have been found to have rates of anaemia in the range 17–48%. Of the older population presenting for surgery, rates of anaemia are higher than quoted in the general population. Two UK studies describing populations presenting for major lower limb joint replacement identified a prevalence of anaemia of 20–25% [4, 5]. A US study of a cohort of hip fracture patients with a mean age of 81.9 years identified anaemia in 40.4% of patients at admission using a single definition of haemoglobin <120 g L^{-1} [6].

A large US veterans cohort study identified pre-operative anaemia in 42.8% of patients presenting for a wide variety of non-cardiac surgery [7]. This study defined anaemia by haematocrit <39%, and comprised 97.7% men, which may partially account for the results. However, another very large US cohort of male and female patients presenting for non-cardiac surgery identified anaemia (again using haematocrit) in 43.7% of the 74,314 over 65-year-olds [8]. While the various definitions of anaemia can make estimates of prevalence difficult, it is clear that a substantial minority of older patients presenting for a wide variety of surgery are anaemic.

Pathophysiology

The causes of anaemia in the elderly can be divided into three broad groups: nutrient deficiency anaemia (principally iron deficiency), anaemia of chronic inflammation (previously termed anaemia of chronic disease) and unexplained anaemia. Conveniently, the proportion of patients falling into each group is about one-third.

Nutrient deficiency anaemia

Anaemia due to deficiencies of iron, B12, or folate, either alone or in combination, accounted for 34.3% of anaemia in the NHANES data, with iron deficiency alone accounting for 16.6% of all anaemia. In industrialised populations, it is rare that dietary deficiency is actually responsible for anaemia, the most frequent cause being chronic gastrointestinal blood loss.

Anaemia of chronic inflammation

Anaemia of chronic inflammation (ACI) accounted for 32.2% of anaemia in NHANES. This is a composite figure, with 8.2% of patients being anaemic in the presence of chronic kidney disease (estimated creatinine clearance

<30 mL min^{-1}) without other comorbidity, 19.7% being anaemic without evidence of renal insufficiency but with other chronic disease, and the remaining 4.3% suffering both renal disease and other disease. Anaemia of chronic inflammation is present in conjunction with a multitude of disease processes, including malignancy, chronic infection, autoimmune disorders and inflammatory conditions. It is usually mild, normochromic and normocytic, with an inappropriately low reticulocyte response, low serum iron and iron-binding capacity, and normal or increased ferritin. Central to understanding the mechanisms of ACI is the hormone hepcidin. Hepcidin is secreted principally by the liver, and inhibits the flow of iron into the plasma from its three principal sources: macrophages involved in the recycling of senescent red blood cells, duodenal enterocytes responsible for absorption of dietary iron and the hepatocellular store. Hepcidin binds to the transmembrane protein transporter ferroportin, and degrades it, preventing iron movement to the bone marrow, thus diminishing erythropoiesis.

Hepcidin is regulated by both iron stores and erythropoiesis. When plasma iron and stored iron are high, hepcidin production is stimulated to decrease intestinal absorption. When plasma and stored iron are low, hepcidin production is suppressed, allowing absorption and free movement of iron. The interaction between erythropoiesis and hepcidin is less well-understood. Erythropoietin (EPO) is not a direct regulator of hepcidin, yet exogenous administration of an erythropoiesis-stimulating agent will cause hepcidin levels to fall, and when the feedback loops are functioning normally, increased erythropoietic activity will also suppress hepcidin.

However, hepcidin production is significantly increased in inflammation or infection. This is principally mediated by interleukin (IL)-6, with the involvement of other cytokine pathways. In chronic conditions of inflammation, this leads to perpetual inhibition of the flow of iron from storage sites to manufacturing sites, with resultant anaemia. Furthermore, inflammatory mediators, including TNFα, IL-1α, IL-1β and reactive oxygen species contribute to the development of ACI by various effects on the regulation of erythropoiesis by EPO. There is inhibition of EPO production in response to anaemia-induced hypoxia, and disruption of the proliferation and differentiation response of erythroid progenitor cells to EPO, with possible EPO resistance [9].

Finally, red cell survival is decreased by cytokines and reactive oxygen species, inducing eryptosis, the death of red cells resulting in phagocytosis by macrophages, further shifting iron into the storage pools.

Unexplained anaemia

The final third (33.6%) of patients in NHANES were labelled as having unexplained anaemia, by which they did not meet definitions for nutrient deficiency, had an adequate serum iron concentration (making ACI unlikely) and did not have chronic kidney disease. It is recognised that this is a rather liberal use of the word 'unexplained', as a proportion of the group will have myelodysplasia, and some early B12 deficiency that was not detectable with simple testing used for this cohort. Others will have a rarer cause of anaemia such as hypothyroidism, spherocytosis, thalassaemia or myeloma that could be identified with further investigation. 'Unexplained' does not therefore equate to 'untreatable', nor should it imply that it is simply a phenomenon associated with ageing homeostatic mechanisms, and therefore less relevant.

Anaemia and outcomes in the elderly

Both anaemia and transfusion of allogeneic red cells have been associated with adverse outcomes, and the potential for anaemia to be a marker of a greater disease burden is frequently raised in discussion. Studies have therefore attempted to control for this using multivariate analysis incorporating other risk factors, and can still demonstrate an independent risk attributable to anaemia.

Community

Cohort studies of patients aged >65 years demonstrate that anaemia, as defined by the WHO criteria, is associated with increased mortality. The US Cardiovascular Health Study cohort showed demographically and fully adjusted hazard ratios (HR) of anaemia for mortality of 1.57 (95% CI: 1.38–1.78) and 1.38 (95% CI: 1.19–1.54) with an 11.2-year follow-up of community-dwelling elderly people [10]. A UK cohort demonstrated similar hazard ratios for men with anaemia (mild anaemia: Hb = 120–129 g L^{-1}, HR = 1.56; severe anaemia: Hb <120 g L^{-1}, HR = 1.87) but although a similar trend was observed, no statistical significance was established for women [1]. Both studies show a 'reverse' J relationship between mortality and haemoglobin level.

More recent analysis of the Cardiovascular Health Study participants demonstrates that haemoglobin decline through the normal range, as well as development of anaemia, is associated with mortality. It is noteworthy that discussion continues in the literature regarding the definition of anaemia in the elderly (as the population used to generate the WHO criteria did not include any over-65s) with studies finding both significant and no significant relationship between haemoglobin at the lower end of the normal range, and outcome.

Anaemia is also associated with a variety of morbidities in older people, being linked with an increase in hospitalisation, poorer physical and cognitive function, development of Alzheimer's and Parkinson's diseases, depression, falls and hip fracture.

The peri-operative period

The initial work on associations between anaemia and surgical outcome originated in cardiac surgery, and studies continue to investigate this population. A recent multinational study of patients undergoing coronary artery bypass grafting identified 4,804 patients of all ages who did not receive a transfusion, and established that patients with a pre-operative haemoglobin of <110 g L^{-1} were at increased risk of adverse postoperative events, the extent of comorbidity amplifying the adverse effects of anaemia [11]. Widening the sphere of observation, two large cohort studies have examined records from National Surgical Quality Improvement Program (NSQIP) databases in the US, of patients undergoing non-cardiac surgery [7, 8]. The earlier study examined >300,000 records of mostly men aged >65 years, and found a rate of anaemia (based on haematocrit) of 42.8%. As haematocrit progressed away from the reference category of 0.45–0.479 in either direction, mortality and cardiac event rates increased. Adjusting for potential confounding variables, and analysing the data using conventional definitions of anaemia and polycythaemia, it established that each percentage point deviation of haematocrit from the normal range resulted in a 1.6% increased risk of adjusted mortality at 30 days.

The later analysis included patients of all ages, such that the mean age was 56.4 years, with 56.7% being female. The baseline rate of anaemia was 30.4%. As would be expected, the anaemic cohort was older, more likely to be non-white, and had higher rates of chronic disease and recent surgery, other than the index event. After adjustment for confounders, anaemia was found to be independently and significantly associated with 30-day mortality and morbidity. Anaemia was associated with higher rates of almost all specific morbidities, with the exception of central nervous system events. The association of anaemia with adverse outcome held across age groups, gender and surgical subspecialty. In common with findings in cardiac surgery, in which anaemia was present concurrently with another recognised risk factor, for example cardiac disease or diabetes, the odds ratio of mortality was higher than if the risk factor was present alone.

These NSQIP data analysis studies are criticised for the heterogeneity of the included populations, with mixing of emergency and elective procedures from many surgical specialties. A more recent secondary analysis of the European Surgical Outcomes Study (EuSOS) also found anaemia to be independently predictive of worse outcomes, though again in a relatively young population (mean age 58) [12]. Smaller studies of focused populations do not unanimously concur that anaemia is an independent risk factor for mortality or morbidity. However, other surgical specialties, for example colorectal surgery, have established the presence of even mild anaemia as an independent risk factor for complications and increased length of stay in a population with mean age of 63.5 years. Meta-analysis of literature reporting on the impact of anaemia on mortality in frailty hip fracture establishes a consistent association between admission haemoglobin and mortality at all measured intervals [13].

Evidence for transfusion thresholds in the elderly

The most expedient method of increasing haemoglobin concentration remains allogeneic red cell transfusion and, when the requirement for surgery is urgent, this may be the only method available.

Parallel to the literature delineating the risk posed by anaemia is a wealth of largely observational data that transfusion is associated with adverse outcomes. Both anaemia and transfusion occur more frequently in populations that are older, and carry a greater burden of comorbidity, and even with statistical manipulation it is difficult to establish with certainty which of anaemia, transfusion or comorbidity is accounting for the subsequent morbidity and mortality.

Allogeneic transfusion can be considered to be a transplant procedure, and as such carries potential for serious harm both from the product itself and the process. There is considerable incentive to avoid transfusion when possible, in terms of both risk management and cost-effectiveness. Guidance produced in 2008 for UK anaesthetists suggests a restrictive use of red cells, with transfusion essential at haemoglobin levels of <50 g L^{-1}, and strongly indicated at <70 g L^{-1}, seeking an endpoint of relative anaemia rather than transfusion to normal haemoglobin levels. A caveat that symptomatic patients may require transfusion outside of these limits allows significant leeway for clinician preference [14]. These triggers are predicated on a physiological understanding of the natural mechanisms that allow tolerance of anaemia, with a large retrospective cohort study of >60-year-old hip fracture patients indicating that 30-day and 90-day mortality was unaltered between groups transfused at Hb <80 g L^{-1}, and those transfused at levels between 80 and 100 g L^{-1} [15]. The TRICC trial [16], often cited as the breakthrough in supportive evidence for restrictive transfusion, evaluated liberal and restrictive strategies of transfusion in critical care patients. It concluded that 'a restrictive strategy of red cell transfusion is at least as effective, and possibly superior to a liberal transfusion strategy in critically ill patients'.

The applicability of this trial to the elderly population needs careful consideration. While there was no upper age limit for entry, the mean age was quite young, with a mean (SD) age of 57.1 (18.1) years in the restrictive group and 58.1 (18.3) years in the liberal group. Mortality rates were statistically different in favour of the restrictive strategy in the under 55s; this was not the case for the older section of the included population, implying equivalence, but not superiority, of a restrictive strategy. Mortality was no different in those with 'clinically significant' cardiac disease in the trial population, but a greater proportion of patients with severe cardiac disease, compared to other disease states, were not enrolled in the study by their attending physician. Consequently, a restrictive strategy is cautioned against in the population with myocardial infarction and unstable angina. Most notably, this trial excluded those with evidence of chronic anaemia, leaving a substantial minority of the elderly ineligible to participate.

Further randomised trials are generally small, but of relevance to the elderly population is a trial of liberal versus restrictive transfusion strategy in a population of elderly people with a history of, or risk factors for, cardiac disease [17]. Patients were recruited to this group if they had a haemoglobin of <100 g L^{-1} after surgery for hip fracture. Primary end points were mortality and functional recovery, assessed as ability to walk independently. Enrolling >2000 patients, with an average age of 81 years, this trial genuinely addressed the geriatric population and again found no difference in primary endpoints between the groups. This work approached the issue with the subtly different emphasis that liberal transfusion may positively improve postoperative recovery, not simply that restrictive strategies do no more harm, and is thus of particular relevance. The caveat for anaesthetists remains that this trial considered transfusion requirements only after surgery was completed, thus it does not address the pre-operative or intra-operative phases of care. Approximately a quarter of both groups had been transfused before randomisation, and this is not followed through the analysis. While very few patients in the liberal group were not transfused (3.3%), 59% of the restrictive group were not transfused after surgery – but may have been before this.

Subsequent to this study, the Cochrane review and meta-analysis of transfusion thresholds have been updated [18]. They include 19 trials with a total of 6264 participants across a variety of surgical, medical and trauma contexts, including children. The transfusion threshold was inconsistent between trials, and for some trials the restrictive trigger equated to a liberal trigger in another setting. Despite this, inclusion in a restrictive transfusion arm did produce a relative risk reduction of transfusion of 39%, with no statistically significant difference in mortality at 30 days nor, when reported, an alteration in length of stay or morbidity. The authors suggest that some adverse events may be associated with liberal transfusion.

Of the 19 studies included in the Cochrane review, only six specifically address the elderly surgical population. These studies have a narrow focus, addressing orthopaedic lower limb procedures including arthroplasty and hip fracture. When this group is separately analysed, the results still support the findings that length of hospital stay and both 30-day and 60-day mortality are not statistically significantly different between restrictive and liberally transfused groups. However, there is a statistically significant (p = 0.05) difference between rates of myocardial infarction, with fewer events in the liberally transfused group. This, in addition to the caution advocated by the Cochrane authors regarding high-risk patient groups such as those with acute coronary syndrome, leaves the issue of anaemia and transfusion in the elderly with cardiovascular disease still open.

Ongoing reporting of literature in this area is starting to fill relevant gaps identified by the Cochrane authors. A study of liberal versus restrictive transfusion policies in older (>55 years) patients receiving mechanical ventilation in critical care has reported recently [19]. This found no difference in major organ dysfunction, duration of mechanical ventilation, infections, cardiovascular complications or mortality and suggests a large-scale trial in this area is feasible.

Other recently published small studies have demonstrated the feasibility of recruiting anaemic patients to trials of transfusion triggers and appropriate separation of groups, while providing information to modify study design for larger randomised controlled trials. As could be expected given the historical literature, the results, based on small numbers, and with some statistically significant differences in group characteristics, are divergent!

Examining the question of the very frail elderly, an abstract presenting a small randomised controlled trial of alternate transfusion triggers in elderly patients with hip fracture admitted from nursing homes, found 90-day mortality to be statistically better in the liberal transfusion group [20]. Extrapolating these results to the UK population will be difficult, as restrictive (Hb = 97 g L^{-1}) and liberal (Hb = 113 g L^{-1}) groups would both be considered liberal by generally accepted UK triggers.

The relative paucity of information generated from randomised, controlled trials of transfusion in the elderly necessitates further consideration of the observational data available, particularly for timeframes other than after surgery, and outcomes other than mortality. One approach to address the conundrum of which type of anaemia, associated comorbidity or transfusion is the causative agent of the observed excess morbidity and mortality, is propensity matching. Akin to multivariate regression analysis, propensity scoring methods attempt to control for variance, balancing the baseline characteristics between treated and untreated groups in observational studies, thus reducing or removing the effect of confounding variables. Large numbers of covariates can be included in a propensity score, and where a pool of potential controls exists, matching extensively can attempt to mimic randomisation for variables that can be measured.

Two publications have used this approach, again accessing the American NSQIP database. One sought to establish the risk of minimal transfusion, i.e. only a single unit of red cells during surgery, compared to no transfusion, working on the assumption that single unit transfusion is most likely to be discretionary. The database excludes children, and only non-cardiac surgery was considered. Over 15,000 cases were identified in which intra-operative single unit transfusion occurred, and approaching 900,000 cases in which no blood was transfused. Unsurprisingly, when unadjusted, the difference in mortality and all measured morbidities was significant between the transfused group and the non-transfused group. After propensity matching for 55 pre-operative variables, and demanding a match to the nearest 0.0001, two groups of 11,855 were identified with a <0.1 standardised difference between groups on all variables. This reveals that transfusion of a single unit of packed red cells significantly increases risks of both mortality and morbidity: wound problems, pulmonary complications, renal dysfunction, and increased length of stay. Cardiovascular and neurological complications, and return to theatre, did not reach significance. While this study was not specifically addressing the elderly, the average age of included patients was 66 years [21].

A second study examined the records of close to 240,000 mostly male veterans seeking the relationship between pre-operative haemoglobin, estimated intra-operative blood loss, and intra-operative transfusion. After propensity score matching, transfusion was associated with a reduction in mortality for those patients with a haematocrit <24% (about 80 g L^{-1}) pre-operatively (odds ratio (OR), 0.60; 95% CI, 0.41–0.87). A reduction in mortality was also seen in patients with higher haematocrits when there was an estimated blood loss of 500–999 mL (haematocrit = 0.30–0.359%; OR, 0.35; 95% CI, 0.22–0.56; haematocrit >0.36% OR 0.78, 95% CI, 0.62–0.97). Conversely, when operative blood loss was estimated at <500 mL, no reduction in mortality was seen in patients with haematocrit between 0.24 and 0.3, and transfusion increased mortality risk in patients with a pre-operative haematocrit of 0.3–0.359 (OR, 1.29; 95% CI, 1.04–1.60). Thus, transfusion harms the mildly anaemic who suffer minimal blood loss. More importantly perhaps, this paper shows that the very anaemic benefit from transfusion as do the moderately anaemic that suffer significant blood loss. This seems to be common sense, but is a fact that has perhaps been lost sight of in the clamour to restrict transfusion.

This pair of propensity-matched studies brings some clarity to areas in which randomisation may be impossible to achieve. However, there are still obvious criticisms of both papers, and this approach will not be suitable to address all the issues surrounding anaemia and transfusion.

Complementary approaches to haemoglobin management

Opportunities to modify patient pathways of peri-operative care to diminish the need for allogeneic transfusion are widespread, and for some years blood management has been advocated. Enacting effective programmes can deliver significant improvements in reduction of rates of anaemia at presentation for surgery, transfusion rates, length of stay and re-admission rates. Fully attributing reduction in bed occupancy to the programme would also suggest very substantial cost savings.

The concept of patient blood management encompasses the pre-operative detection and management of anaemia, the minimisation of blood loss, restrictive transfusion practices and the harnessing of physiological capacity to tolerate anaemia, for example normovolaemic haemodilution and oxygen supplementation. Specific guidelines exist for some surgical specialties [22]. However, understanding core generic principles and the application of these to current local practice and circumstance would seem as likely to bring improvement.

Key to the management of pre-operative anaemia is the separation of the patient who is iron deficient from the patient with iron sequestration, i.e. those with ACI. Practically, this means that patients identified with anaemia should proceed to have either serum ferritin or transferrin saturation measured. Treatment options for iron deficiency and ACI are iron alone, erythropoietic stimulant, or both. Oral iron has a place in the treatment of iron deficiency. However, intravenous iron should be the first choice where there is limited time for optimisation or the patient is intolerant or non-compliant. Logically, oral iron will be ineffective in the patient with ACI, hence a diagnostic trial of intravenous iron in these patients may be successful, or provide confirmation of the necessity to proceed to the use of erythropoietic stimulants with iron supplementation.

References

1. Mindell J, Moody A, Ali A, Hirani V. Using longitudinal data from the health survey for England to resolve discrepancies in thresholds for haemoglobin in older adults. *British Journal of Haematology* 2013; **160**: 368–376.
2. Eisele L, Durig J, Broecker-Preuss M, et al. Prevalence and incidence of anemia in the German Heinz Nixdorf recall study. *Annals of Hematology* 2013; **92**: 731–737.
3. Guralnik JM, Eisenstaedt RS, Ferrucci L, et al. Prevalence of anemia in persons 65 years and older in the United States: evidence for a high rate of unexplained anemia. *Blood* 2004; **104**: 2263–2268.
4. Saleh E, McClelland DB, Hay A, et al. Prevalence of anaemia before major joint arthroplasty and the potential impact of preoperative investigation and correction on perioperative blood transfusions. *British Journal of Anaesthesia* 2007; **99**: 801–808.
5. Kotzé A, Carter LA, Scally AJ. Effect of a patient blood management programme on preoperative anaemia, transfusion rate, and outcome after primary hip or knee arthroplasty: a quality improvement cycle. *British Journal of Anaesthesia* 2012; **108**: 943–952.

6. Halm EA, Wang JJ, Boockvar K, et al. Effect of perioperative anemia on clinical and functional outcomes in patients with hip fracture. *Journal of Orthopaedic Trauma* 2004; **18**: 369–374.

7. Wu W-C, Schifftner TL, Henderson WG, et al. Preoperative hematocrit levels and postoperative outcomes in older patients undergoing noncardiac surgery. *Journal of the American Medical Association* 2007; **297**: 2481–2488.

8. Musallam KM, Tamim HM, Richards T, et al. Preoperative anaemia and postoperative outcomes in non-cardiac surgery: a retrospective cohort study. *Lancet* 2011; **378**: 1396–1407.

9. Macciò A, Madeddu, C. Management of anemia of inflammation in the elderly. *Anemia* 2012. http://dx.doi.org/10.1155/2012/563251 (accessed 9/1/2015).

10. Zakai NA, Katz R, Hirsch C, et al. A prospective study of anemia status, hemoglobin concentration, and mortality in an elderly cohort. *Archives of Internal Medicine* 2005; **165**: 2214–2220.

11. Kulier A, Levin J, Moser R, et al. Impact of preoperative anemia on outcome in patients undergoing coronary artery bypass graft surgery. *Circulation* 2007; **116**: 471–479.

12. Baron DM, Hochrieser H, Posch M, et al. Preoperative anaemia is associated with poor clinical outcome in non-cardiac surgery patients. *British Journal of Anaesthesia* 2014; **113**: 416–423.

13. Potter LJ, Doleman B, Moppett IK. A systematic review of pre-operative anaemia and blood transfusion in patients with fractured hips. *Anaesthesia* 2015; **70**: 483–500.

14. Association of Anaesthetists of Great Britain & Ireland, 2008. Blood Transfusion and the Anaesthetist: Red Cell Transfusion 2. http://www.aagbi.org/sites/default/files/red_cell_08.pdf (accessed 9/1/2015).

15. Carson JL, Duff A, Berlin JA, et al. Perioperative blood transfusion and postoperative mortality. *Journal of the American Medical Association* 1998; **279**: 199–205.

16. Herbert P, Wells G, Blajchman M, et al. A multicenter, randomized, controlled clinical trial of transfusion requirements in critical care. *New England Journal of Medicine* 1999; **340**: 409–417.

17. Carson JL, Duff A, Berlin JA, et al. Liberal or restrictive transfusion in high-risk patients after hip surgery. *New England Journal of Medicine* 2011; **365**: 2453–2462.

18. Carson JL, Carless PA, Herbert PC. Transfusion thresholds and other strategies for guiding allogeneic red blood cell transfusion. *Cochrane Database of Systematic Reviews* 2012, issue 4, Art no. CD002042.

19. Walsh TS, Boyd JA, Watson D, et al. Restrictive versus liberal transfusion strategies for older mechanically ventilated critically ill patients: a randomized pilot trial. *Critical Care Medicine* 2013; **41**: 2354–2363.

20. Gregersen M, Borris LC, Damsgaard EM. A liberal blood transfusion strategy improves survival in nursing home residents with hip fracture. *European Geriatric Medicine* 2013; **4**: S106.

21. Ferraris VA, Davenport DL, Saha SP, Austin PC, Zwischenberger JB. Surgical outcomes and transfusion of minimal amounts of blood in the operating room. *Archives of Surgery* 2012; **147**: 49–55.

22. Goodnough LT, Maniatis A, Earnshaw P, et al. Detection, evaluation, and management of preoperative anaemia in the elective orthopaedic surgical patient: NATA guidelines. *British Journal of Anaesthesia* 2011; **106**: 13–22.

CHAPTER 8

Organ Donation and the Anaesthetist

Dale Gardiner[1,2], Neal Beckett[3], Paul Townsley[1] and Helen Fenner[1]

[1]Nottingham University Hospitals NHS Trust, Nottingham, UK
[2]NHS Blood and Transplant, Bristol, UK
[3]Musgrave Park Hospital, Belfast, UK

Key points

- The number of potential organ donors each year in the UK is only around 6,000.
- There are four types of donation possible from a human body.
- Substantial progress in organ donation and transplantation has occurred in the UK since 2008.
- There is a robust and comprehensive ethical, legal and professional framework for organ donation in the UK.
- Advice is given for the theatre anaesthetists involved in living or deceased organ recovery.

When Joseph Murray carried out the world's first kidney transplant in 1954, it looked like the world was going to change, and it has – but only by one donor at a time. Meanwhile, the number of patients on the transplantation waiting list has continued to grow, far outstripping the number of donors. The World Health Organization has called for national self-sufficiency in transplantation to protect the vulnerable from exploitation. While we await a transforming breakthrough in xenotransplantation or the technology for laboratory-grown organs, patients die: three per day in the UK. It is only through the generosity of donors and their families that the gift of life has been given to so many. Anaesthetists have, since transplantation began, acted as essential guardians of this gift. We, more than any other group, are the clinicians entrusted with recognising futility, diagnosing death, honouring wishes of the deceased and their

---

AAGBI Core Topics in Anaesthesia 2015, Edited by William Harrop-Griffiths, Richard Griffiths and Felicity Plaat.

family, and facilitating donation and transplantation in theatre. This chapter explores the current policy and practice in UK organ donation and the essential role that anaesthetists, with a special focus on theatre anaesthetists, continue to play.

Living kidney donation, because of the differences compared to deceased donation, will be discussed separately and the first part of this chapter concentrates, unless stated otherwise, on deceased donation.

Organ donation policy

Types of organ and tissue donation

Table 8.1 outlines the four types of donations that are possible from a human body. Donation after circulatory death (DCD) or non-heart-beating organ donation was the original type of deceased organ donation prior

Table 8.1 The four types of donation

Type	Requires	Donated
Living	Consenting living donor; donating a non-vital part of the human body.	• Kidneys (1,114 transplants) • Liver lobe (32 transplants) • Lung lobe (0) – internationally performed • Bone marrow • Blood (~2 million donations)
Tissue donation	Deceased in mortuary ideally within 4 h after death; donation usually within 24 h.	• Cornea donors (3,146) • Heart valves • Skin • Bone and ligaments
Donation after brainstem death (DBD)	Organ recovery in theatre with circulation maintained in a mechanically ventilated patient after death has been confirmed using neurological criteria.	780 donors resulted in transplants: • Kidney (1,321) • Liver (727) • Pancreas (203) • Intestine (26) • Lung (182) • Heart (193)
Controlled donation after circulatory death (DCD)*	Organ recovery commencing in theatre ideally within a maximum of 15 min after death has been confirmed using circulatory criteria following the withdrawal of life-sustaining treatment.	540 donors resulted in transplants: • Kidney (821) • Liver (153) • Pancreas (43) • Lung (35)

Source: NHS Blood and Transplant Statistics 2013–2014.
*See text for a description of uncontrolled DCD.

to the acceptance of neurological criteria for human death that allowed donation after brain(stem) death (DBD) or heart-beating organ donation. In DCD, warm ischaemia begins as the circulation fails; organ viability for transplantation likewise rapidly falls (within 20 min for the liver) and this form of donation was effectively abandoned in the UK for 25 years. It was because of the unmet need on the transplant waiting list and because families in intensive care were advocating organ donation for their relatives who were not brainstem dead that programmes of DCD recommenced.

Controlled DCD usually involves a mechanically ventilated patient with predominantly overwhelming single organ failure, usually the brain, where a prior decision has been made to withdraw life-sustaining treatment because this is to the patient's overall benefit. The independent UK Donation Ethics Committee recommends that two senior doctors be involved in making the decision to withdraw life-sustaining treatment. If there is a clinical expectation that the circulation will cease imminently upon the withdrawal of life-sustaining treatment (within 4 h), DCD may be possible. If consent for organ donation is obtained during discussion with the family by the Specialist Nurse for Organ Donation (SNOD), a surgical retrieval team is mobilised. Withdrawal only commences once the surgical team is prepared in theatre and recipients for the organs have been identified. The SNOD supports the family throughout this process. The time from family consent to withdrawal is usually a minimum of 12 h and this can occasionally lead some families to revoke their consent. DCD accounts for 40% of all deceased organ donation in the UK, which makes the UK a world leader in this form of donation. As a result of the warm ischaemic organ damage that occurs in DCD, transplantation outcomes are mixed when compared to DBD organs. Apart from single centre novel practice in Denver, USA; Sydney, Australia; and now in Cambridge, UK; there are as yet no DCD national heart programmes. Livers and pancreases have worse outcomes in DCD but the long-term results for kidneys are equivalent. Lung DCD results are either equivalent or perhaps even superior to DBD lungs, as the lack of a coning phase leading to brainstem death means that there is less neurogenic pulmonary injury, though outcome results are still limited to small numbers (see Donation after circulatory death later in the chapter).

Uncontrolled DCD is a form of donation carried out in France, Spain and historically in a few centres in the UK. Currently, there is a pilot in process in Edinburgh. It involves rapid organ recovery following an unexpected death, hence the term 'uncontrolled' compared to a planned, 'controlled' withdrawal of life-sustaining treatment. The usual case involves failed cardiopulmonary resuscitation either in the emergency department or in the community.

The UK organ donation potential

Many are surprised – and the public is generally ignorant of the fact – that the number of potential organ donors each year in the UK is only around 6,000. This is because organ viability fails so quickly when the circulation ceases, that unless circulation is maintained until organ recovery (DBD) or a surgical team is ready to recover the organs rapidly after the circulation ceases (DCD), no donation can occur; although tissue donation may be possible. In effect, this means that only patients whose lungs are being mechanically ventilated have any realistic possibility of becoming organ donors, and highlights the vital role anaesthetists have in identifying and referring all ventilated patients where extubation and end-of-life care is planned. Figure 8.1 outlines annual deaths in the UK and the potential for organ donation.

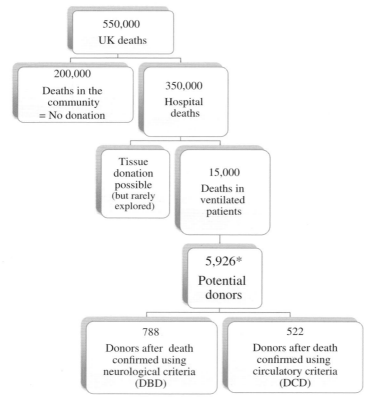

Figure 8.1 Deaths in the UK and the organ donation potential. *Donation data from the 2013–14 NHS Blood and Transplant Potential Donor Audit. A potential donor for the purposes of this figure is a patient who may be deceased using neurological criteria but is yet to be tested (1,787 patients), or had treatment withdrawn in the ICU or emergency department in 2013–14, where death was anticipated within 4 h, and had no absolute medical contraindications to solid organ donation (4,139 patients).

Overall, the number of patients who can be confirmed as deceased using neurological criteria (brainstem dead) is decreasing as improved road safety, neuroradiological early coiling of subarachnoid haemorrhages and decompressive craniectomies have benefited many patients.

The UK organ donation report card

Five years ago, there were no Clinical Leads for Organ Donation, no SNODs, no chairs of donation committees and a donation rate among the lowest in the industrialised world (see Figure 8.2). It is not that efforts had not been tried before. In spite of a British Medical Association report in 2000 and a Department of Health report in 2003, by 2005 the UK had the lowest number of donors on record. Then, in 2008, the Organ Donor Taskforce reported and, for the first time, there was government backing for real action.

Of the 14 recommendations made, the recommendation to make donation a local concern has probably had the greatest impact. Previously there

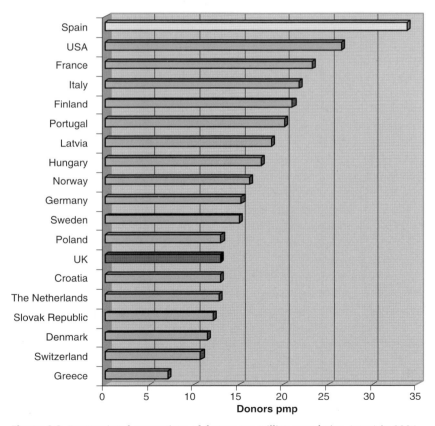

Figure 8.2 International comparison of donors per million population (pmp) in 2006. *Source*: Dr Paul Murphy, NHS Blood and Transplant, http://www.irodat.org

were 18 coordinator teams across the country. These were replaced by 190 local donation teams, all supporting organ donation in their hospital. This model had made Spain the world leader in organ donation. In Spain, intensive care doctors are appointed to full-time organ donation roles. The UK model for local donation teams is different (and less well funded) and consists of

- Clinical Lead for Organ Donation (CLOD), usually an intensive care doctor reimbursed for 4 h per week.
- Specialist Nurse for Organ Donation (SNOD): a full-time nurse (part-time in smaller hospitals) employed by NHS Blood and Transplant who is assigned to a hospital on an honorary contract and attached to the ICU.
- Non-clinical Chair of the hospital Organ Donation Committee.
- Organ Donation Committee, reporting directly to the hospital board and ideally, in large hospitals, having direct theatre and theatre anaesthetic representation, not just intensive care.

A second successful impact deriving from the Taskforce's recommendations is the effort that has been made to resolve outstanding legal, ethical and professional issues in organ donation. This has ensured that all clinicians are supported and are able to work within a clear and unambiguous framework of good practice, including the establishment of the independent, UK Donation Ethics Committee. These issues are explored later, but it is clear that there has been wide consensus and high-level supportive publications produced in a short period of time.

The consensus view from ethicists, legal experts and professional bodies such as the General Medical Council, the National Institute for Health and Care Excellence and the Intensive Care Society, is that donation should not be viewed as something that is inflicted upon patients and families. Rather, it should be considered to be a fundamental component of end-of-life care and should not be denied to patients because they are dying in the wrong place or in the wrong way.

The Taskforce recommendations were implemented as part of a 5-year plan with a goal of increasing donation by 50% over this period. On 31 March 2013 the 5 years concluded and, in the UK, donation had increased by the targeted 50%. For 3 years, more deceased donations and transplants were carried out than ever before and, for the first time, the transplant waiting list has decreased (Figure 8.3). However, the increase in donation was mostly accounted for by a 153.5% increase in DCD compared to only a 15.8% increase in DBD (Figure 8.4). Kidney recipients have been the biggest beneficiaries of the 50% increase. Whereas those waiting for other organs, particularly hearts, which only come from DBD, have benefited much less: at the end of the 5 years, the UK remains

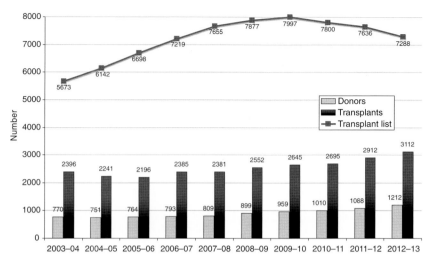

Figure 8.3 Deceased donors, transplants and the transplant waiting list 2003–13.
Source: Dr Paul Murphy, NHS Blood and Transplant, http://www.irodat.org

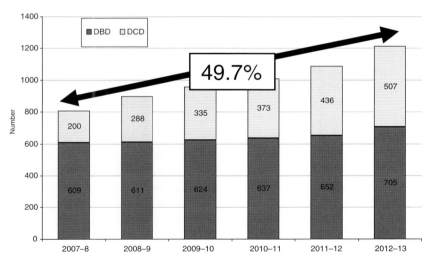

Figure 8.4 Deceased organ donors in the UK from the benchmark 2007–2008 financial
year to the end of the Organ Donor Taskforce 5-year goal of a 50% increase by 31
March 2013. The largest rise is in donation after circulatory death (DCD): 153.5%,
compared to donation after brainstem death (DBD): 15.8%.
Source: Dr Paul Murphy, NHS Blood and Transplant, http://www.irodat.org

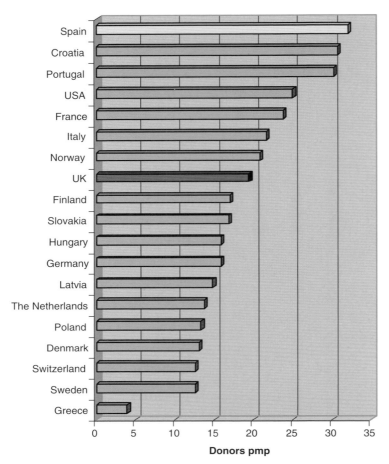

Figure 8.5 International comparison of donors per million population (pmp) in 2012. *Source*: Dr Paul Murphy, NHS Blood and Transplant, http://www.irodat.org

only a middle-order donation country (Figure 8.5). One league table the UK consistently tops is family refusal (Figure 8.6). Wales has enacted soft, presumed consent (deemed consent) legislation (commencing December 2015), but the effect this will have on family refusal is unknown and it remains ethically challenging, particularly in DCD.

Scientific, ethical and legal issues in deceased donation

The diagnosis of death

Deceased organ donation first requires the patient to be confirmed as being deceased. This obvious statement is encapsulated in what Robertson coined the 'Dead Donor Rule' [1], though its implications can be narrowed to 'prohibiting only the killing of patients for organ donation' or broadened to

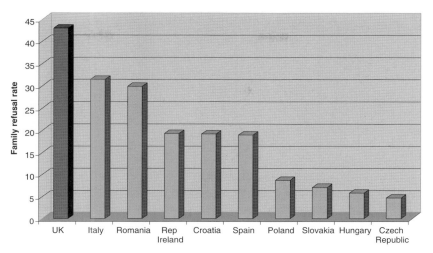

Figure 8.6 European comparison of family refusal rate (as percent).
Source: Dr Paul Murphy, NHS Blood and Transplant adapted from the Global
Observatory on Donation and Transplantation,
http://www.transplant-observatory.org/Pages/home.aspx

'procedures for organ donation should not be initiated while the patient is
still alive', depending on which philosophical discourses one favours. What
is clear worldwide is that publications and debate on the diagnosis of death
and deceased donation are closely intertwined. This is not necessary, as
the 2008 Academy of Medical Royal Colleges *Code of Practice for the Diagnosis and Confirmation of Death,* quite progressively outlined diagnostic criteria
for death suitable for all patients, irrespective of organ donation.

The declaration of death is in most countries the legal responsibility of
a medical practitioner. However, dying is a process that affects different
functions and cells of the body at different rates. Doctors must decide at
which moment along this process there is permanence, and death can be
appropriately declared. Our understanding and the criteria we use may
have evolved, but our duty remains the same: to make a timely diagnosis of death while avoiding any diagnostic errors – an obligation medical
professionals cannot and should not abdicate.

There is growing medical consensus in a unified concept of human death.
All human deaths involve the permanent loss of the capacity for consciousness, combined with the permanent loss of the capacity to breathe. Death
is therefore a result of the permanent loss of these essential capacities in
the brain, and specifically in the brainstem. Three sets of criteria can be
used to establish the permanent loss of these capacities and thus diagnose
human death (Figure 8.7). The most appropriate set of criteria to use is
determined by the circumstances in which the medical practitioner is called
upon to diagnose death. In the community and where death may have

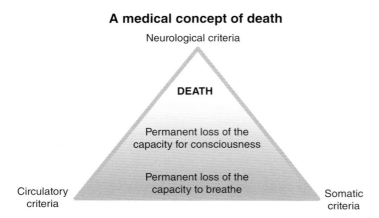

Figure 8.7 The three criteria for diagnosing human death.

occurred by overwhelming trauma or many hours previously, somatic criteria, being features visible on external inspection of the corpse, for example decapitation and decomposition, will reliably indicate the loss of these two essential capacities. When death is more recent and especially within a hospital setting, death is usually diagnosed by the use of circulatory criteria after cardiorespiratory arrest. It is only within the critical care environment, in which mechanical ventilation is used, that the diagnosis of death using neurological criteria is applied (Table 8.2). The Intensive Care Society has endorsed forms for the diagnosis of death using neurological criteria [2].

A summary of the current published best practice, ethical, legal and professional guidance

Human Tissue Acts (2004 and 2006)

The Human Tissue Act 2004 covering England, Wales and Northern Ireland [3] and the Human Tissue (Scotland) Act 2006 [4] set out the legislative requirements for seeking consent and authorisation to donation, both living and deceased.

Primacy of the prior expressed consent or authorisation of the patient is established by the Acts. Registration on the Organ Donor Register equals consent or authorisation for the purposes of donation, with the family having no legal right of veto, though in practice donation is never forced upon a dissenting family in the UK.

The Human Transplantation (Wales) Bill 2013 introduces deemed (soft opt out) consent into Wales from December 2015. The law will only apply in Wales for Welsh residents over 18 years of age. Families will still be approached to ascertain if the potential donor may have objected to donation.

Table 8.2 Essential components for the diagnosis of death using circulatory criteria following cardiorespiratory arrest and neurological criteria in patients in ventilated coma

Components of the diagnosis of death using circulatory criteria	Components of the diagnosis of death using neurological criteria
A clear intention not to attempt cardiopulmonary resuscitation in order to restore circulatory, and therefore cerebral, function.	An established aetiology capable of causing structural damage to the brain which has led to the permanent loss of the capacity for consciousness combined with the permanent loss of the capacity to breathe.
An examination and observation period to confirm continuous apnoea, absent circulation and unconsciousness, after which the likelihood of spontaneous resumption of cardiac function will have passed. Five minutes is accepted in the UK.	An exclusion of reversible conditions capable of mimicking or confounding the diagnosis of death using neurological criteria.
The prohibition at any time after the diagnosis of death of any intervention that might restore cerebral blood flow by any means.	A clinical examination of the patient that demonstrates profound coma, apnoea and absent brainstem reflexes.

Academy of Medical Royal Colleges Code of Practice for the Diagnosis and Confirmation of Death (2008)

This was the successor to previous versions and updated the Code of Practice published in 1976, 1979, 1983 and 1998 for the diagnosis of death using neurological criteria. It was notable for being the first Code of Practice to provide guidance on the diagnosis of death following cardiorespiratory arrest (circulatory criteria), and the first code of practice to remove organ donation considerations from the guidance.

Legal guidance from all four UK jurisdictions on DCD (2009–2011)

DCD may be in the person's interests [5–7]:
- By maximising the chance of fulfilling the donor's wishes about what happens to them after death.
- By enhancing the donor's chances of performing an altruistic act of donation.
- By promoting the prospects of positive memories of the donor after death.

The following steps are permissible to facilitate DCD [5–7]:
- Delaying withdrawal of life-sustaining treatment.
- Changing the patient's location.
- Maintaining physiological stability.

Joint professional statement from the Intensive Care Society and the British Transplantation Society (2010)

This document [8]:

1 Stated professional support for DCD.
2 Gave professional support for admission to ICU purely for organ donation.
3 Defined suitability criteria for donation.
4 Provided guidance for treatments before and after death.

General Medical Council Guidance: 'Treatment and care towards the end of life' (2010)

This guidance [9] includes the following statements:

- If a patient is close to death and their views cannot be determined, you should be prepared to explore with those close to them whether they had expressed any views about organ or tissue donation, if donation is likely to be a possibility
- You should follow any national procedures for identifying potential organ donors and, in appropriate cases, for notifying the local transplant coordinator [specialist nurse – organ donation].

Joint professional statement from the College of Emergency Medicine and the British Transplantation Society (2011)

This statement [10] provided:

- Professional support for the robust identification of potential donors in the emergency department.
- Professional support for managing organ donation from the emergency department if admission to ICU is not possible.

Independent UK Donation Ethics Committee (2011)

Provides guidance on roles, responsibilities, and conflicts of interest [11]:

- Early referral to the SNOD is acceptable.
- Two senior clinicians should make the decision that life-sustaining treatment should be withdrawn.
- Care should be in an appropriate environment and provided by staff with the appropriate skills and experience to deliver the end-of-life care plan.
- After death, it is acceptable for the treating clinician to take actions necessary to facilitate donation, for example tracheal re-intubation.

NICE Guidance (2011)

This guidance [12] set out the expected standard of practice applicable in England, Wales and Northern Ireland and recommended:

- Triggered referral if there is a:
  - Plan to withdraw life-sustaining treatment.
  - Plan to perform brainstem testing.

○ Catastrophic brain injury (early referral), defined as the absence of one or more cranial nerve reflexes, for example one fixed pupil and a Glasgow Coma Scale score ≤ 4 that is not explained by sedation.

• While assessing the patient's best interests clinically, stabilise the patient in an appropriate critical care setting while the assessment for donation is performed. For example, an adult intensive care unit or in discussion with a regional paediatric intensive care unit.

• A collaborative approach to the family for organ donation involving:
  ○ A SNOD.
  ○ A local faith representative if appropriate.

College of Emergency Medicine Best Practice Guidance for End of Life Care (2012)

This guidance [13] stated that:

• Organ and tissue donation should be considered as a usual part of end-of-life care in the emergency department.

• Emergency department staff should consider organ donation from all patients that are expected to die, whose trachea is intubated and whose lungs are ventilated.

• Referrals should be made via specialist nurses in organ donation.

Organ donation practice for the theatre anaesthetist

Identifying and referring potential donors

While the majority of potential organ donors are identified in ICUs, in 2012 14% were identified in the emergency department. However, more than two-thirds of patients dying in the emergency department who are potential organ donors are still not having organ donation explored as an option in their end-of-life care, and are effectively denied the option of organ donation regardless of their wishes. Anaesthetists have a unique opportunity and responsibility to identify and refer potential donors, particularly those patients whose tracheas are intubated and whose lungs are ventilated outside intensive care and are undergoing tracheal extubation for end-of-life care.

Some anaesthetists have questioned the appropriateness of early referral to the specialist nurses. The unequivocal ethical and professional support for this duty has been outlined above. The independent UK Donation Ethics Committee is very clear: 'There is no ethical dilemma if the treating clinician wishes to make contact with the SNOD at an early stage while the patient is seriously ill and death is likely, but before a formal decision has been made to withdraw life-sustaining treatment. [Benefits] include establishing whether there are contra-indications for organ donation. Other practical and organisational factors might be relevant – if the SNOD is based at a distant location, then early contact can help to minimise distressing delays for the family.'

A significant number of complaints to NHS Blood and Transplant every year are from relatives where organ donation was not explored for their loved one, whereas complaints regarding inappropriate exploring of organ donation are extremely rare. Early referral is no different to checking there is a bougie on hand for a rapid sequence induction; it is preparing for plans B and C, even if B and C never occur.

Before approaching any family regarding organ donation:
- Always **PLAN** the family approach with the SNOD.
- **DO NOT** raise organ donation with the family until it is clear that they have understood and accepted their loss or they raise the topic themselves.

Donation after brainstem death

Many anaesthetists will go through their training without ever being involved in organ retrieval, so unfamiliarity can bring apprehension. Transplant and retrieval teams do not routinely provide an anaesthetist, although they may have a physiologist in attendance. Reassuringly, the transplant and retrieval teams are supportive of the theatre staff and anaesthetist and will commonly guide and support them through the process. Good communication is essential.

The primary role of the anaesthetist is to ensure optimal tissue perfusion and protection of the organs during surgery by optimising the donor's haemodynamic status and gas exchange until cross-clamping of the aorta. This is often straightforward, but the anaesthetist should be prepared to maintain organ perfusion in a potentially unstable patient.

The following guidelines are designed to assist anaesthetic staff in pre-operative and intra-operative management. A donor optimisation bundle is available from NHS Blood and Transplant [14]. The specific drugs used during surgery should be discussed with the SNOD before patient transfer to theatre and with the transplant and retrieval teams. It is useful to have a briefing with the team before the start of surgery to ensure a unified plan.

The primary challenges for the anaesthetist are the following:
- Unstable haemodynamics, hypothermia, diabetes insipidus.
- Persisting spinal reflexes, both neuromuscular and autonomic.
- ECG changes, arrhythmias and decreased myocardial compliance.

Cardiovascular management

- Donors may be dehydrated from attempts to control intracranial pressure or from diabetes insipidus.
- Restoring an effective circulating volume should be the first priority.

- Give a rapid 3–5 mL kg^{-1} 'fluid challenge' of a balanced crystalloid or colloid and carefully assess the response.
- Mean arterial pressure should be maintained between 60 and 80 mmHg.
- Ideally, cardiac output monitoring should be used.
- When hypotension persists and signs of vasodilatation are present, restoration of vascular tone with vasopressin may be the most effective measure to restore blood pressure (dose: 0.5–4 units h^{-1}). Usually this has already been started in the ICU.
- Often, inotropic support is required; the choice of catecholamine will be dictated by retrieval team preferences and invasive monitoring results.
- Dopamine is now more frequently considered to be an appropriate first line drug with dobutamine as an alternative.
- High dose catecholamine therapy, especially with noradrenaline, is associated with poor graft function and the chance of cardiac retrieval may be decreased.
- When the response to catecholamine infusion is inadequate, consider a trial of intravenous hydrocortisone 50–100 mg.
- Some cardiovascular instability should be anticipated during placement of slings around the inferior vena cava and aorta, and during handling of the heart and large blood vessels.
- Variations in blood pressure may be controlled with vasodilators, high dose opiates such as fentanyl and volatile anaesthetics.
- Cardiac performance may also be affected by hormonal changes, and some teams may ask for thyroid hormone supplementation in the form of a tri-iodothyronine (T3) bolus and infusion. This is usually given as an infusion of 3 μg h^{-1}.

Respiratory management
- Lung recruitment manoeuvres are important.
- Use 'lung protective' ventilation: tidal volumes 6–8 mL kg^{-1} with optimal PEEP to allow for minimum oxygen requirement.
- Maintain a PaO$_2$ > 8.0 kPa (SpO$_2$ = 92–95%).
- Peak inspiratory pressures should be <30 cm H$_2$O.
- Maintain PaCO$_2$ at 4.7–6 kPa unless oxygenation is an issue and then permissive hypercapnia is allowed so long as arterial pH > 7.25.

Fluid management
- Avoid a positive fluid balance and hypernatraemia.
- Correct any electrolyte abnormalities, especially of potassium, magnesium, phosphate and calcium.
- Monitor urine output and maintain at 1–2 mL kg^{-1} h^{-1}
- If urine output is >4 mL kg^{-1} h^{-1}, consider diabetes insipidus and treat with DDAVP or vasopressin.

- Monitor blood glucose and start an insulin infusion to maintain glucose at 4–10 mmol.L^{-1}.
- Ensure that the patient is 'grouped and saved' in case blood products are needed during organ recovery. Local transfusion triggers apply.

Medication administration

A long-acting non-depolarising neuromuscular-blocking drug of the anaesthetist's choice should be given before the surgical procedure after consultation with the retrieval team.

When dissection is complete, heparin 300 units kg^{-1} (20,000–25,000 units) is usually given and the various intravascular cannulae are then placed for organ perfusion. The surgeon will advise the anaesthetist on when to give heparin.

Most transplant teams use methylprednisolone (15 mg kg^{-1} up to 1 g) and a broad-spectrum antibiotic. The timing of administration varies; commonly it is given at the start of donor surgery.

The process of organ recovery

- The SNOD will usually contact the anaesthetist and operating theatre staff to arrange a suitable theatre time and to advise them about the equipment required.
- The largest operating room available should be used, subject to other needs of the donor hospital.

Equipment

- Standard monitoring including invasive pressures (arterial and central venous pressure) and temperature should be used. It is preferable that use of the femoral artery is avoided.
- At least one large bore intravenous cannula should be placed before theatre for rapid volume replacement
- Ideally, a means of temperature management placed underneath the patient before transfer to limit surgical interference.

Positioning

- Check body positioning with transplant teams – the possible positions they may choose are
  - Arms by the side.
  - Arms outstretched to 90 degrees.
  - Arms hyperextended and taped above the head.
- Supine with both arms hyperextended above the head gives best access for both the surgical teams and the anaesthetist. Usual concerns about the brachial plexus injury do not apply.

Donation after circulatory death

When only intra-abdominal organs are being recovered, the role of the theatre anaesthetist is predominantly logistic. The surgical team needs a vacant theatre and may wait up to four hours after withdrawal of life-sustaining treatment occurs, provided warm ischaemia (SpO_2 < 70% or systolic blood pressure < 50 mmHg) has not started. The surgical team is usually self-sufficient with support from the SNOD, but will require a 'runner' to help them access equipment and set up suction in an unfamiliar hospital.

In the UK, the withdrawal of life-sustaining treatment usually occurs in the ICU, so that patient and family care can continue uninterrupted, but if the ICU is some distance from theatre it may occur in the theatre post-anaesthesia care unit or in an anaesthetic room. Warm ischaemia is damaging to organ viability, so when the deceased donor is moved onto the operating table, the surgeons must open and gain access to the organs rapidly to allow cold perfusion and organ preservation.

Lung DCD

Evidence is emerging that DCD lungs transplanted following cardiorespiratory arrest produce a survival equal or superior to lung DBD. It is well recognised that brain death and the process of coning can cause an acute lung injury. There are several mechanisms by which this may occur:

- Uncontrolled sympathetic nervous system activation causes an increase in pulmonary capillary hydrostatic pressure. The resulting trauma to the capillary-alveolar membrane increases capillary permeability and leads to neurogenic pulmonary oedema.
- Alongside this process, there is a profound inflammatory response within the lungs, which further increases capillary permeability. This may be neurologically mediated or as a direct result of capillary trauma.
- A later, prolonged period of neurogenic hypotension follows the hypertensive crisis prolonging the systemic inflammatory response; this may worsen the acute lung injury.

Compared to the lung insult after brain death, the lungs appear to be significantly less injured by the warm ischaemia that occurs after cessation of the circulation. This difference is likely to contribute to the different outcomes seen after transplant.

Role of anaesthetist during lung DCD

Safe lung DCD requires some specific input from the anaesthetic team:

- Patient transfer to theatre. Transfer must be rapid to minimise warm ischaemia time. In hospitals in which the operating theatre is a significant distance from the ICU, thought should be given to withdrawal of treatment in an appropriate location nearer to the theatre, for example theatre complex post-anaesthesia care unit.

- Re-intubation and airway protection. If the patient's trachea is extubated on withdrawal of life-sustaining treatment, it will be necessary to re-intubate the patient's trachea before organ recovery to prevent aspiration and soiling with gastric contents. It is not advised to inflate the lungs at the time of intubation, as this is considered a resuscitative measure and risks restoring spontaneous circulation. Confirming correct tube placement may be difficult because of this, plus the fact that even if the lungs were inflated, there would be no end-tidal carbon dioxide present due to the absence of cardiac output. If a difficult tracheal intubation is anticipated, thought must be given to the chosen method of intubation or not extubating in the first place.
- Early inflation of the lungs with oxygen. Successful lung DCD requires oxygenation to reduce warm ischaemic damage. However, consensus guidance by the Intensive Care Society and British Thoracic Society in 2010 recommends that this should be performed no earlier than 10 min after the onset of asystole. Inflation should be performed using a single positive pressure recruitment manoeuvre, for example continuous positive airway pressure (CPAP) at 40 cmH_2O for 45 seconds followed by maintenance of CPAP at 5 cmH_2O. Under no circumstances should the patient's lungs be cyclically ventilated at this time.
- Ongoing support of the thoracic retrieval team. Lung recovery will usually take place after abdominal organ retrieval, as the lungs are remarkably resilient to warm ischaemia once inflated with oxygen. When lung retrieval starts, the lungs will undergo cold perfusion. Gentle ventilation will be required to distribute the perfusate evenly. If there is any concern that this may restore circulation, the thoracic surgeons may isolate the cerebral circulation using a cross-clamp across the arch of the aorta.

Living kidney donation (living donor renal transplant nephrectomy)

In an attempt to meet demand, there has been a threefold increase in living donor renal transplants in the last 10 years. More than one third of all renal transplants are from living donors (Table 8.1). Although there has been some consensus on the approach to management by transplant surgeons and nephrologists, the approach to anaesthesia has tended to develop on a largely ad hoc basis in local centres.

Legal framework

All kidney transplants performed from living donors must comply with the requirements of the primary legislation (Human Tissue Act 2004 and Human Tissue (Scotland) Act 2006) [3, 4]. This legislation established a regulatory body, the Human Tissue Authority, to oversee and control the working of the Act. The Human Tissue Authority must ensure informed consent, absence of inducement or coercion and assessment by an independent assessor.

The primary legislation allows the following types of living donation for kidney transplantation:

- Directed donation – donation to a specific recipient:
  - Genetically related.
  - Emotionally related.
  - Paired: donor incompatible with the potential recipient – matched with another donor/recipient pair.
  - Pooled: more than two donor/recipient pairs are involved in exchange.
- Altruistic, non-directed: kidney is donated by a healthy person with no relationship with recipient.

Ethical considerations

There is a wide range of complex moral issues associated with this area of transplantation. Key ethical principles involved include:

- Altruism
- Autonomy
- Beneficence
- Non-maleficence
- Dignity
- Reciprocity

None of the benefits to a recipient justify living donation unless the interests of the donor are given primacy. A living donor nephrectomy is morally acceptable when carried out with informed consent, freely given.

Surgical considerations

Living donor renal transplantation has advantages:

- Availability of senior staff
- Known quality of organ to be transplanted
- Ability to plan daytime surgery and optimise recipient factors
- Increased graft survival

Surgical techniques for living donor nephrectomy:

- Open
- Laparoscopic
- Hand assisted laparoscopic

Laparoscopic factors:
- Lower analgesic requirements
- Decreased blood loss and trauma
- Earlier resumption of food intake
- Shorter hospital stay
- More technically demanding
- Comparable complication rates

The left kidney is usually preferred, due to the greater length of the left renal vein.

Anaesthetic management

Pre-operative assessment
It is possible to be healthy but not suitable for donation, for example single kidney. All potential donors require a full pre-operative anaesthetic, medical and psychological assessment. Renal function is assessed to ensure that the donor will have sufficient kidney function after donation and sufficient graft function in the recipient. Any risk of latent or current infection in the donor needs to be identified.

Most donors are ASA physical status I or II, being deemed 'complicated' if older with multiple comorbidities, body mass index >30 kg m^{-2}, vascular renal abnormalities, requiring a right nephrectomy or refusing blood products. Hypertension is not a contraindication if diastolic pressure is controlled (<85 mmHg) but nephrectomy may worsen the condition. The only relative contraindications are aged <18 years or having diabetes mellitus. Written consent is sought before admission, and reconfirmed on admission.

Peri-operative management
- Theatre planning to minimise ischaemic time
- Consultant anaesthetist and surgeon
- WHO safety checklist carried out
- Wide bore intravenous access
- Maintain normothermia
- Non-invasive blood pressure monitoring unless specific indication for invasive monitoring
- Central venous catheter: aim for positive fluid balance, set CVP target after clamp release; most centres aim for 12–15 cm H_2O
- Near full lateral position with extension break at the waist
- Thrombo-embolism prophylaxis, for example, pneumatic compression devices, graduated stockings, low molecular weight heparin
- Combination of general anaesthesia with tracheal intubation and regional analgesia

- Fluids: maintain positive fluid balance with crystalloid
- Give intravenous heparin before arterial clamping
- Maintain perfusion pressure with intravenous fluid and dopamine
- Maintain urine output >80 mL h^{-1} – mannitol 0.5 g kg^{-1}
- Analgesia options:
    - Transversus abdominis plane block
    - Paravertebral block
    - Local infiltration, for example, port sites by surgeon
    - Infusion of local anaesthetic by wound catheter
    - Patient-controlled analgesia with an opiate drug
    - Non-steroidal analgesic drugs if not contra-indicated – avoid if serum creatinine >170 mmol L^{-1}

Additional considerations
- Hand assisted nephrectomy – routine chest physiotherapy and prokinetics help reduce postoperative chest infections and paralytic ileus.
- A transplant unit should undertake at least 20–30 living donor operations per year.
- Donor and recipient operations may be carried out sequentially or using dedicated, parallel theatres. Aim to minimise cold ischaemic time and unforeseen problems with the recipient.
- Living kidney donors are classified as 'medium risk' patients for deep venous thrombosis and pulmonary embolism. Donors with history of thrombo-embolism or thrombophilia are 'high risk'. NICE-approved thromboprophylaxis policy should be followed.
- There is no evidence to support the use of prophylactic antibiotics in donor surgery. Some centres use a single dose at induction.
- Blood transfusion is rarely needed. All donors should be 'grouped and saved'.
- Hydration begins with an overnight infusion of fluid. Some units use intravenous mannitol or loop diuretics during surgery and trans-oesophageal Doppler to guide fluid replacement.
- Early postoperative pain is the most frequent complaint. The laparoscopic technique avoids the need for an epidural, with patient-controlled analgesia and regional anaesthesia techniques enabling early mobilisation. Frequently pain is often due to abdominal incision, port-site pain, diaphragmatic irritation, ureteric colic or pelvic organ pain. A small number of patients may require referral to a pain clinic.

Mortality and morbidity
The most common causes of death after living donation are pulmonary emboli, hepatitis and cardiac events. The risk of peri-operative mortality

is around 0.03%. Analysis of UK registry data has shown the major morbidity rate after laparoscopic donor nephrectomy to be 4.5–5.1% for open nephrectomy [15] and includes re-operation, bleeding, bowel obstruction, bowel injury, hernia, thrombo-embolic events, pneumothorax, ileus, chest infection and delayed discharge (1–2%). Up to 3–5% of donors get chronic wound pain. An increase in serum creatinine normalises within 1 month. Micro-albuminuria persists in 20%, while long-term renal function remains at 75%.

Acknowledgements

With thanks to Dr Paul Murphy (National Clinical Lead for Organ Donation, NHS Blood and Transplant) for the use of his adapted figures.

References

1. Robertson JA. The dead donor rule, *Hastings Center Report* 1999; **29**(6): 6–14.
2. Intensive Care Society. Guidelines & Standards. http://www.ics.ac.uk/ics-homepage/guidelines-and-standards/ (accessed 21/4/2015).
3. Human Tissue Act 2004. http://www.legislation.gov.uk/ukpga/2004/30/contents (accessed 21/4/2015).
4. Human Tissue (Scotland) Act 2006. http://www.legislation.gov.uk/asp/2006/4/contents (accessed 21/4/2015).
5. Legal issues relevant to non-heartbeating organ donation. Department of Health, 2009. http://www.dh.gov.uk/en/Publicationsandstatistics/Publications/Publications PolicyAndGuidance/DH_108825 (accessed 21/4/2015)
6. Guidance on legal issues relevant to donation following cardiac death. Scottish Government, 2010. http://www.scotland.gov.uk/Publications/2014/10/3139/5 (accessed 21/4/2015).
7. Legal issues relevant to donation after circulatory death (non-heart-beating organ donation) in Northern Ireland. Department of Health, Social Services and Public Safety, 2011. http://www.dhsspsni.gov.uk/donation-after-circulatory-death-legal-guidance-march-2011.pdf (accessed 21/4/2015).
8. Donation after Circulatory Death. British Transplantation Society, 2010. http://www.bts.org.uk/Documents/Guidelines/Active/DCD%20for%20BTS%20and%20ICS%20FINAL.pdf (accessed 21/4/2015).
9. Treatment and care towards the end of life: good practice in decision making. General Medical Council, 2010. http://www.gmc-uk.org/guidance/ethical_guidance/end_of_life_care.asp (accessed 21/4/2015).
10. *The Role of Emergency Medicine in Organ Donation*. Royal College of Emergency Medicine/British Transplantation Society, 2011. www.rcem.ac.uk/code/document.asp?ID=6175 (accessed 12/5/2015).
11. An Ethical Framework for Controlled Donation after Circulatory Death. UK Donation Ethics Committee, 2011. http://www.aomrc.org.uk/doc_view/9322-an-ethical-framework-for-controlled-donation-after-circulatory-death (accessed 21/4/2015).

12. Organ donation for transplantation: improving donor identification and consent rates for deceased organ donation. NICE, 2011. http://guidance.nice.org.uk/CG135 (accessed 21/4/2015).

13. The College of Emergency Medicine. *End of life care for patients in the Emergency Department*. Best Practice Guidance (February 2012).

14. Donor optimisation. http://www.odt.nhs.uk/donation/deceased-donation/donor-optimisation (accessed 21/4/2015).

15. Hadjianastassiou VG, Johnson RJ, Rudge CJ, Mamode N. 2509 living donor nephrectomies, morbidity and mortality, including the UK introduction of laparoscopic donor surgery. *American Journal of Transplantation* 2007; **7**: 2532–2537.

Recommended reading

Diagnosis of Death and Organ Donation. *British Journal of Anaesthesia* 2012; **108**(suppl.): i1–i121. http://bja.oxfordjournals.org/content/108/suppl_1.toc (accessed 21/4/2015).

For a good review of the UK Organ Donation Policy with some controversial suggestions: British Medical Association: *Building on Progress: Where next for organ donation policy in the UK?* http://bma.org.uk/-/media/files/pdfs/working%20for%20change/improving%20health/organdonation_buildingonprogressfebruary2012.pdf (accessed 21/4/2015).

NHS Blood and Transplant Microsite for Professionals (includes brain death forms, donor optimisation guidance and forms): Organ Donation and Transplantation. http://www.odt.nhs.uk

UK Guidelines for Living Donor Kidney Transplantation: Compiled by a Joint Working Party of The British Transplantation Society and The Renal Association – http://www.bts.org.uk

Author's (DG) website – http://www.clodlog.com

CHAPTER 9

Postoperative Cognitive Dysfunction: Fact or Fiction?

Irwin Foo
Western General Hospital, Edinburgh, UK

> ### Key points
>
> - Postoperative cognitive disorders are common, and the elderly are particularly susceptible.
> - Postoperative cognitive dysfunction (POCD) remains a research finding, with no consensus on diagnostic criteria, but with identified negative clinical outcomes, for example impairment of activities of daily living, premature loss from the workforce and increased mortality.
> - POCD is by definition a transient phenomenon with recovery within 1 year of surgery.
> - There is no difference in the incidence of POCD when general anaesthesia is compared with regional anaesthesia plus sedation.
> - The most consistent risk factors for POCD are advanced age and poor cognitive reserve.
> - Strategies shown to decrease the incidence and impact of POCD include fast-track techniques and anaesthesia care with bispectral index and cerebral oxygen saturation optimisation.
> - Routine screening of the older patient for the presence of cognitive impairment before surgery is important to identify patients at risk of postoperative cognitive decline.

After surgery and anaesthesia, patients may notice deterioration in memory and a decreased ability to handle intellectual challenges. Some may complain that they are 'just not the same' for weeks or months after their surgical procedure. This decline in cognitive functioning after surgery tends to be subtle and can occur even after seemingly uncomplicated anaesthesia and minor surgery. Although these changes can occur in all age groups, the elderly appear to be more susceptible. Despite being anecdotally identified by both patients and healthcare professionals, there exists debate about

AAGBI Core Topics in Anaesthesia 2015, Edited by William Harrop-Griffiths, Richard Griffiths and Felicity Plaat.
© 2015 The Association of Anaesthetists of Great Britain and Ireland (AAGBI).
Published 2015 by John Wiley & Sons, Ltd.

the existence of POCD as a distinct clinical entity and its extent. The term 'POCD' was popularised after a series of studies in the 1990s, but it remains a research phenomenon. It has yet to gain an International Classification of Disease Diagnostic (ICD-10) code or a Diagnostic and Statistical Manual of Mental Disorders (DSM-IV) code because of the lack of consensus on diagnostic criteria. This chapter aims to explore the issues surrounding this controversial clinical condition and its relevance to surgical patients.

Cognition and postoperative cognitive disorders

Cognition literally means 'to know' and includes perception, memory and information processing that allows us to acquire knowledge, solve problems and plan for the future. These are mental processes essential for everyday living and should not be confused with intelligence. Patients complain when these processes are disrupted and often describe their dysfunction in terms of memory loss, poor concentration, a slowing down of executive function and abstract thought.

Postoperative cognitive conditions found in patients can be categorised into three conditions: delirium, POCD and dementia. These conditions are distinguished by the timings of their presentation and duration of symptoms (Figure 9.1). Historically, delirium and POCD were seen as manifestations of the same disease entity, but more recent research suggests that despite similarities, these two conditions should be considered as separate conditions [1]. Table 9.1 illustrates the differences found in these two

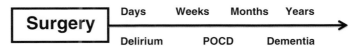

Figure 9.1 Timeline in postoperative cognitive conditions.

Table 9.1 Differences between delirium and postoperative cognitive dysfunction

	Delirium	POCD
Onset	Hours to days	Weeks to months
Characteristic of onset	Acute	Subtle
Duration	Days to weeks	Weeks to months
Consciousness	Altered but with lucid intervals	Normal
Concentration and attention	Impaired	Impaired
Reversibility	Yes	Yes, but can be prolonged

conditions. Dementia, on the other hand, consists of multiple cognitive deficits, of which memory impairment is essential for diagnosis, along with significant problems with social activities and behaviour to the extent that it interferes with daily function and independence. Although there are anecdotal reports in which catastrophic cognitive deterioration has occurred after anaesthesia and surgery, resulting in a diagnosis of dementia, they are rare, poorly studied and will not be considered further here.

Delirium

Delirium is well defined. According to the ICD-10 code, it is an 'aetiologically non-specific organic cerebral syndrome characterised by concurrent disturbances of consciousness and attention, perception, thinking, memory, psychomotor behaviour, emotion and the sleep-wake schedule. The duration is variable and the degree of severity ranges from mild to very severe'. Frequently complicating the course of hospitalised patients (the incidence varies depending on the patient population and ranges from 25% to 60% in elderly patients), its onset is most often within the first 3 days after surgery. Typically the condition fluctuates throughout the day, with periods in which the patient is disorientated and confused. It may be associated with an altered level of consciousness and although it tends not to persist beyond 1 week, it is now recognised that it may be present for weeks. It is important to appreciate that delirium is a behavioural syndrome and is diagnosed by observing the patient. The most commonly used test is the Confusion Assessment Method, which provides a standardised rating of delirium that has been validated against the DSM-IV. It is essentially a bedside tool with high interobserver reliability and both high sensitivity (93–100%) and high specificity (89–100%) [2].

Delirium is frequently characterised into subtypes: hyperactive (agitation and restlessness are predominant symptoms: 15% of cases), hypoactive (lack of responsiveness, slow or absent movement and slowed speech are predominant: 35%), mixed picture (vacillates between hyperactive and hypoactive symptoms: 26%) and a recent addition: subsyndromal (presence of some but not all symptoms or cannot be classified into any subtype: 24%). Although delirium is not the main focus of this chapter, it is important to emphasise that delirium may persist beyond 1 week and both subsyndromal and hypoactive delirium are both easily missed if not tested for formally. Both may complicate the interpretation of tests used to detect early POCD, often carried out 1 week after surgery.

Postoperative cognitive dysfunction

Unlike delirium, POCD is less well-characterised and has no agreed universal definition. It can be usefully defined as a research finding of deterioration in neurocognitive testing that requires pre-operative and postoperative tests to diagnose. As it is a more subtle condition, diagnosis can be challenging. Furthermore, POCD affects a wide variety of cognitive domains, for example memory, information processing and executive functioning, and patients differ in the domains most affected. Typically, patients complain of deterioration in memory, poor ability to carry out complex tasks or to multitask, and impairment in language skills, for example comprehension and word finding.

Interest in this area began with Bedford's observation in 1955 [3] in which he reported that 7% of elderly post-surgical patients developed dementia after general anaesthesia. This was based on his personal observations and by questioning patient relatives, hospital staff and others. No form of formal neuropsychological testing was carried out. He concluded that 'operations on elderly patients should be confined to unequivocally necessary cases only'. However, this was not universally accepted, as a later study by Simpson et al. using standardised neuropsychological testing found that any deterioration could be readily explained by other causes [4]. Subsequent studies attempting to document the presence of POCD failed to detect any dysfunction beyond a short time after surgery.

These early studies served to illustrate the difficulties in measuring cognitive changes in patients in the postoperative setting. Apart from the use of low-sensitivity tests to detect cognitive changes, there are other issues that had to be addressed. First, both pre-operative and postoperative cognitive testing is essential in diagnosing POCD. It is the change from the baseline pre-operative test that is the important factor, as each patient is acting as their own control. Baseline testing should represent the patient's best results and it is therefore important to take into account any medications that the patient is taking and to rule out any pre-existing neuropsychiatric disorder, for example depression, which can impair cognitive function greatly. Furthermore, a person's cognitive performance varies, i.e. there are natural fluctuations in performance, and both the environment in which the testing is carried out and the personnel conducting the test can influence results. Second, there is a natural age-related decline in both cognitive function and practice effects that has to be accounted for in the tests used, along with test–retest reliability of the individual tests themselves. Therefore, the use of an age-appropriate control group is essential, and the tests themselves should have parallel versions to minimise the learning effect. Third, as different domains may be affected to different extents in individual patients experiencing cognitive change, the use of single tests is no longer appropriate, and test batteries are now recommended and should be standardised. Fourth, cognitive testing should be carried out at baseline and after surgery at a time when the patients are unlikely to be under the influence of postoperative analgesics or other medications that may interfere with cognition.

The International Study of Postoperative Cognitive Dysfunction Group

A series of studies carried out in the late 1990s by the International Study of Postoperative Cognitive Dysfunction (ISPOCD) group were designed to circumvent the methodological difficulties in assessing cognitive function after surgery. A test battery of four neuropsychological tests (Table 9.2) was selected to assess learning, memory and executive function (concentration, processing speed), along with tests for depression, activities of daily living and subjective assessment of cognitive change. This test battery takes approximately 30 min to complete and, to account for practice effects and natural fluctuations of test results, a control group of volunteers (not undergoing surgery) were also tested at the same time points as the post-surgical patients.

The diagnosis of POCD was based on Z-scores, for which the practice effect found in the control population was corrected. The Z-score is a dimensionless unit that indicates how far an individual's test performance deviates, in terms of standard deviation (SD), from the average performance of the control sample. Postoperative cognitive dysfunction was arbitrarily defined as a Z-score of ≥ 2 and is therefore based on a statistical cut-off rather than the magnitude of change in the pre-test to post-test scores of individual patients.

Table 9.2 Neuropsychological tests used in the ISPOCD studies

Test	What does it measure?
Visual verbal learning test Ability to memorise 15 words in three consecutive trials, and their recall after 15–25 min.	Immediate recall and short-term working memory.
Concept shifting task 16 standardised circles with numbers, letters or both, crossed out in a specific preset pattern.	Visual conceptual and visuomotor skills.
Stroop colour word test Naming the colour of the words printed in different colour ink to the word they represent, for example the word 'red' is printed in blue ink rather than red and the correct answer is 'blue'.	Selective attention, cognitive flexibility and processing speed as an indicator of executive functioning.
Letter digit coding test Test shows nine letters with an allocated number to each letter. Patient fills in the missing number in rows of horizontal lines of letters with an empty box underneath. Patient completes as many as possible in 1 minute.	Speed of processing and combination of domains: visual scanning, perception, visual memory and motor functions.

In the landmark ISPOCD1 study by Moller et al., using the criteria discussed above, the incidence of POCD was quantified in 1,218 patients aged >60 years after non-cardiac surgery [5]. They also recruited 321 controls who did not undergo an operation. They found an incidence of POCD of 25.8% in patients tested 7 days after surgery (which they termed 'early POCD') and in 9.9% after 3 months ('late POCD'), compared to a control incidence of approximately 3% at both time points. Furthermore, in a subset of patients followed up for 1–2 years, the incidence of POCD was found to be the same as in the control sample (10.4% vs 10.6%) but, due to the small number of control subjects (n = 47), the confidence intervals were wide [6]. Therefore, the majority of patients with POCD improved over time. Interestingly, only three patients (~ 1%) had POCD at all three postoperative test sessions, which led the authors to conclude that POCD is reversible in the majority of patients but may persist in 1% of patients.

Other studies conducted by the ISPOCD investigators themselves or using ISPOCD methodology produced the following results:

- Early POCD (1 week after surgery) is common and similar in incidence in any age group after major non-cardiac surgery performed under general anaesthesia.
- Late POCD (3 months after surgery) is less common than early POCD, but with a clear relationship with age (7% in those aged >60 years and 14% in those aged >70 years).
- Early POCD is more common after major surgery (25.8%) than after minor surgery (6.8%), and is higher in inpatients. The difference in late POCD is much smaller (6.6% vs 9.9%).
- No difference was found between general and regional anaesthesia (with sedation), although there was a trend towards higher early POCD with general anaesthesia.
- There was a higher mortality after surgery in patients who had both early and late POCD (five times more likely to be dead 1 year after surgery) or just late POCD.
- Early POCD was found to predispose to an increased risk of being unemployed and on benefit payments.
- In patients who were found to have late POCD, memory disturbance was prominent, and patients with executive function disturbance had more severe functional impairment in terms of instrumental activities of daily living, for example the ability to handle finances and be responsible for their own medications.

In a systematic review on POCD after non-cardiac surgery performed by Newman et al., the authors suggested that the majority of studies in this field were underpowered to draw firm conclusions – an estimated sample size for each group of 199 was required to assess POCD adequately after surgery [7]. Out of 46 studies reviewed, only five had a group sample size of this magnitude, and the majority came from the ISPOCD group of investigators. This supported the robustness of the results from this group of investigators.

Although this discussion has so far focused on POCD after non-cardiac surgery, it is becoming clear that off-pump cardiac surgery produces a similar effect on cognitive function to surgery using cardiopulmonary bypass. This suggests that factors other than cerebral embolic damage resulting from cardiopulmonary bypass are contributing to the POCD seen in this group of patients. Thus, there may be more similarities than differences between these two patient groups.

The case against POCD

POCD is not a recognised disease or syndrome. Opponents of POCD as a distinct entity maintain that it is a statistical abnormality with little clinical basis, and is essentially a research finding. It has also been suggested that the term 'POCD' has outlived its usefulness and should no longer be used, as it only serves to increase anxiety among older surgical patients and may impact on their decision to proceed with surgery.

A persisting problem with POCD lies in the interpretation of test results. Different batteries of neuropsychological tests have been used (>70 different tests) and different thresholds have been set by different investigators to define POCD. For example, the threshold set by the ISPOCD investigators is a decline of 2 SDs based on those derived from control data. Other investigators have used 1.0 or 1.5 SD as the criteria. This makes comparison of test results difficult, and the less rigorous the criteria, the higher the incidence of POCD. In addition, this method of reporting does not take into account the floor and ceiling effects of the individual tests. Typically, patients who do really well on the pre-operative test will not change much because they have reached the maximal achievable correct answers (ceiling effect) and the same is true for the poorest performers (floor effect). In addition, there is often a gap between the test results and patient's self-perceived cognition, raising questions about the specificity and sensitivity of the tests, or alternatively whether the patient overestimates postoperative cognitive problems. Furthermore, POCD should not be diagnosed as a categorical condition, i.e. presence versus absence, as cognition is a continuous measure and should be quantified on a scale such that changes in scores may be analysed.

Many studies in this field had no control group and in others the control group was not well matched to the surgical group. As already mentioned, a control group is necessary to quantify the practice effect with repeated testing. However, as the control group tends to be recruited from healthy volunteers, there is a tendency for this group to be performing above average in cognitive tests. This may well result in an overestimation of the practice effect. Very few studies include delirium testing as part of their assessment. Delirium may persist beyond 1 week and is easily missed, especially the hypoactive and subsyndromal types, unless actively sought. It is conceivable that some patients diagnosed with early POCD when tested at 1 week after surgery may still be suffering from delirium that was undetected. In this situation, the test results would be inappropriately poor. Furthermore, it is possible that at 1 week after surgery, residual pharmacological effects from analgesics may have contributed to the impairment in cognitive performance.

When patients present for surgery, they may have pre-existing cognitive decline. Information about the trajectory of patients' cognitive status before surgery is helpful to prevent the misdiagnosis of POCD, as the apparent decline in neuropsychological tests could merely reflect a pre-existing trend (Figure 9.2a). In a retrospective study conducted by Avidan et al. [8], three groups were identified from participants tested annually in an Alzheimer's Disease Research Centre: those who had non-cardiac surgery, a major illness or neither (control group). The battery of neuropsychological tests performed was comprehensive and, using sophisticated statistical methods, the authors were able to assess the subjects' cognitive function before and after non-cardiac surgery or major illnesses. The study found that neither non-demented nor mildly demented participants in the database had accelerated long-term decline in cognitive function after surgery or major illness when compared with matched controls. Therefore, this suggested that neither surgery nor major illness were independent risk factors associated with long-term cognitive decline. However, as the assessments were carried out annually, it cannot rule out the possibility of an early cognitive decline (at 1 week and 3 months) after surgery, followed by subsequent recovery (Figure 9.2b).

Evered et al. studied the incidence of pre-existing cognitive impairment in 152 patients aged >60 years scheduled for elective total hip replacement [9]. They found that 20% of patients had evidence of pre-existing cognitive impairment, and that this figure was much higher (55%) in those aged over 80 and importantly, all these patients had normal activities of daily living. The conclusion that can be drawn from this study is that we are routinely anaesthetising and operating on a large proportion of older patients whose brains are already significantly compromised.

The possibility that POCD is a transient phenomenon is supported by a recent study by Kline et al., who used both clinical and neuroimaging data from participants in the Alzheimer's Disease Neuroimaging Initiative [10]. They investigated whether participants in the database who had undergone

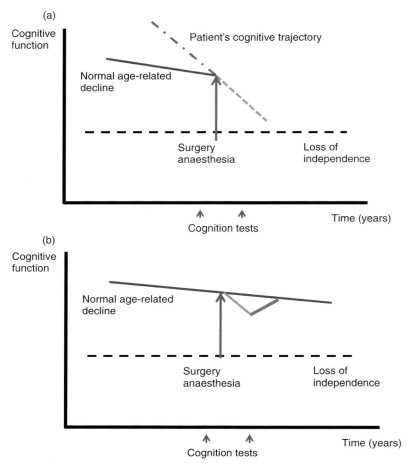

Figure 9.2 Cognitive trajectory and apparent decline in neuropsychological tests.
(a) An illustration of a situation where the patient demonstrates an apparent decline in
cognitive function when tested before and after surgery. However, if this patient's
cognitive trajectory was known beforehand, this may represent a pre-existing trend
that is independent of anaesthesia and surgery. (b) An illustration of a transient decline
in cognition after surgery followed by subsequent recovery.

surgery had brain and cognitive trajectory changes similar to those in a
matched non-surgical cohort. They found that surgical patients on average demonstrated greater cortical and hippocampal volume loss compared
with the non-surgical cohort at the first follow-up visit (~ 6 months after
surgery). Furthermore, those who had baseline mild cognitive impairment
(MCI – defined as impairment in one or more cognitive domains greater
than would be expected for a person's age, but otherwise functionally intact
and capable of living independently), met the criteria for POCD at the first
follow-up visit after surgery. However, at subsequent follow-up visits, both

the neuro-imaging and cognitive performance tests were no longer different from the non-surgical patients. This is in keeping with Avidan's study conclusion that surgery alone is not associated with long-term cognitive decline, but also supported the notion that POCD is a transient event triggered by surgery.

Is POCD fact or fiction?

The term POCD remains controversial. It is primarily a research finding and is variably defined, as there is no consensus on its diagnostic criteria. Although POCD may be regarded as a clinical myth, the diagnosis of POCD has clear negative clinical outcomes: it is a predictor of impairment of activities of daily living, premature loss from the workforce and death.

Major illness or surgery and anaesthesia can result in a transient worsening of cognition that improves with time. This is measurable by neuropsychological tests and is reflected in reversible anatomical changes in specific brain regions. Although it can affect all ages, it is more common and longer lasting in the elderly. Age is the most consistent factor associated with POCD. It is becoming evident that patients with poor cognitive reserve, i.e. patients with MCI, may be at greater risk of worsening cognition after surgery. Furthermore, as about 10–40% of older patients living in the community may have MCI, it is likely that these patients will present for anaesthesia and surgery. Risk factors for POCD are summarised in Table 9.3.

Table 9.3 Risk factors for postoperative cognitive dysfunction

Early POCD (tested 7 days after surgery)
- Increasing age
- Increasing duration of anaesthesia
- Cardiac and orthopaedic surgery
- Major operations, redo operations
- Postoperative infection
- Respiratory complication
- Lower educational level

Late POCD (tested 2 weeks or more after surgery)
- Increasing age
- Lower educational level
- Pre-existing mild cognitive impairment
- Previous cerebral vascular accident
- High alcohol intake or alcohol abuse
- Early POCD
- Postoperative delirium

Patients, and especially older patients, and their carers should be made aware of this transient decline in cognition, as it may impact on early post-discharge activities such as taking medications and self-care. They should be reassured that there is improvement with time and resuming full general activities, particularly exercise, may hasten its resolution. The danger with older patients is that once their confidence is eroded and independence is lost, it is more difficult to return them to their pre-operative state, for example once a decision to go to a supervised facility is taken, it is unlikely to be reversed.

As cognitive impairment occurs after major illness as well as after surgery, should the term POCD be abandoned? At present, I would argue against this as it serves to remind us how vulnerable the brain is in the peri-operative period, and persuades us to institute measures to minimise its occurrence. Interestingly, it has been suggested that POCD may even be MCI or a subset of MCI by another name as these two conditions bear so many similarities [11]. Of course, this requires further investigation and confirmation, but if they turn out to be similar entities, then POCD would change from being a research diagnosis to a clinically recognised condition of decreased cognitive reserve that is unmasked by anaesthesia and surgery.

What can be done about POCD?

Suggested pathophysiological mechanisms causing POCD include the postoperative stress response, neuro-inflammation, disturbed sleep architecture, poor pain control and opioid usage, and neurotoxicity from anaesthetic drugs, especially volatile anaesthetics. There is evidence in *in vitro* and animal studies that suggests these factors are important, but there are very few clinical correlates, for example all volatile anaesthetics are neurotoxic *in vitro* and animal models have demonstrated that sevoflurane and isoflurane can both induce apoptosis and worsen amyloid β peptide oligomerisation and deposition, a process associated with cognitive dysfunction with Alzheimer's disease. A recent pilot study in patients even suggested that there may be differences between volatile agents, with desflurane causing less cognitive disturbance than isoflurane when neuropsychological testing were carried out 7 days after surgery [12].

As anaesthesia and surgery exacerbate cognitive decline, it is prudent to keep both as minimally invasive and as short as possible. Two recent strategies appear to be promising in decreasing the impact of POCD. Fast-track techniques that focus on early mobilisation, multimodal opioid-sparing analgesia and early discharge have been demonstrated by Krenk et al. to be associated with a decrease in the incidence early POCD 1 week after hip or knee replacement when compared to previous studies (9.1% vs 25% from the ISPOCD group) [13]. Optimised peri-operative care and early discharge from hospital were believed to be the main reasons for the decrease in the incidence of POCD. Another strategy that decreased the incidence of POCD was that used by Ballard et al., in which intra-operative bispectral index values were maintained at 40–60, and cerebral oxygen saturation was both monitored and optimised with blood pressure manipulation, adjustment of inspired oxygen concentration, end-tidal carbon dioxide concentration and blood transfusion [14].

Furthermore, as the elderly are at particular risk of postoperative cognitive impairment, there is a need to screen them routinely for the presence of pre-operative cognitive impairment. The tests and criteria used for diagnosis should be compatible with those established for the diagnosis of MCI. Routine testing would allow a direct comparison of post-surgical results with the well-established longitudinal databases in the general population of MCI and cognitive trajectory. In the meantime, we should investigate patients who say that their cognition is impaired at 3 months after surgery and refer them for neurocognitive testing even if they had no pre-operative tests. They may have decreased cognitive reserve compatible with a diagnosis of MCI that has been unmasked by anaesthesia and surgery.

The future

As the population ages, more elderly patients will be presenting for surgery and anaesthesia. Efforts to improve the physiology of an ageing body may put additional stress on the brain, especially if there is already decreased cognitive reserve. Identifying this group of patients is important, as they are likely to be compromised after surgery. To facilitate this, a consensus should be reached on which tests are the most suitable both before and after surgery, and strategies to minimise POCD instituted based on test results. The relationship between POCD and MCI should be elucidated, along with the role of surgery and anaesthetic drugs in the pathogenesis of POCD.

References

1. Krenk L, Rasmussen LS. Postoperative delirium and postoperative cognitive dysfunction in the elderly – what are the differences? *Minerva Anesthesiologica* 2011; **77**: 742–749.
2. Silverstein JH, Deiner SG. Perioperative delirium and its relationship to dementia. *Progress in Neuro-Psychopharmacology & Biological Psychiatry* 2013; **43**: 108–115.
3. Bedford PD. Adverse cerebral effects of anaesthesia on old people. *Lancet* 1955; **266**: 259–263.

4. Simpson BR, Williams M, Scott JF, Crampton Smith A. The effects of anaesthesia and elective surgery on old people. *Lancet* 1961; **278**: 887–893.
5. Moller JT, Cluitmans P, Rasmussen LS, et al. Long-term postoperative cognitive dysfunction in the elderly: ISPOCD1 study. *Lancet* 1998; **351**: 857–861.
6. Abildstrom H, Rasmussen LS, Rentowl P, et al. Cognitive dysfunction 1–2 years after non-cardiac surgery in the elderly. *Acta Anaesthesiologica Scandinavica* 2000; **44**: 1246–1251.
7. Newman S, Stygall J, Hirani S, et al. Postoperative cognitive dysfunction after non-cardiac surgery. A systematic review. *Anaesthesiology* 2007; **106**: 572–590.
8. Avidan MS, Searleman AC, Storandt M, et al. Long-term cognitive decline in older subjects was not attributable to non-cardiac surgery or major illness. *Anesthesiology* 2009; **111**: 964–970.
9. Evered LA, Silbert BS, Scott DA, et al. Pre-existing cognitive impairment and mild cognitive impairment in subjects presenting for total hip joint replacement. *Anesthesiology* 2011; **114**: 1297–1304.
10. Kline RP, Pirraglia E, Cheng H, et al. Surgery and brain atrophy in cognitively normal elderly subjects and subjects diagnosed with mild cognitive impairment. *Anesthesiology* 2012; **116**: 603–612.
11. Silbert B, Evered LA, Scott DA, et al. Anesthesiology must play a greater role in patients with Alzheimer's disease. *Anesthesia & Analgesia* 2011; **112**: 1242–1245.
12. Zhang B, Tian M, Zhen Y, et al. The effects of isoflurane and desflurane on cognitive function in humans. *Anesthesia & Analgesia* 2012; **114**: 410–415.
13. Krenk L, Rasmussen LS, Kehlet H. Delirium in the fast-track surgery setting. *Best Practice & Research Clinical Anaesthesiology* 2012; **26**: 345–353.
14. Ballard C, Jones E, Gauge N, et al. Optimised anaesthesia to reduce postoperative cognitive decline (POCD) in older patients undergoing elective surgery, a randomised controlled trial. *PLoS ONE* 2012; **7**: 1–9.

Further reading

Avidan MS, Evers AS. Review of clinical evidence for persistent cognitive decline or incident dementia attributable to surgery or general anesthesia. *Journal of Alzheimer's Disease* 2011; **24**: 201–216.

Grape S, Ravussin P, Rossi A, et al. Postoperative cognitive dysfunction. *Trends in Anaesthesia and Critical Care* 2012; **2**: 98–103.

Krenk L, Rasmussen LS, Kehlet H. New insights into the pathophysiology of postoperative cognitive dysfunction *Acta Anaesthesiologica Scandinavica* 2010; **54**: 951–956.

Nadelson MR, Sanders RD, Avidan MS. Perioperative cognitive trajectory in adults. *British Journal of Anaesthesia* 2014; **112**: 440–451.

CHAPTER 10

Pre-Operative Anaemia: Should We Worry?

Robert Kong

Brighton and Sussex University Hospitals NHS Trust, Brighton, UK

Key points

- The World Health Organization definition of anaemia is a haemoglobin concentration <13 g.l^{-1} in men and <12 g.l^{-1} in women.
- Pre-operative anaemia is associated with increased postoperative morbidity and mortality.
- Large observational studies strongly suggest that pre-operative anaemia is an independent risk factor for adverse outcomes.
- A low pre-operative haemoglobin concentration predisposes patients to increased peri-operative blood transfusion and contributes to postoperative morbidity.
- Iron deficiency, the commonest cause of pre-operative anaemia, is treatable.
- Pre-operative anaemia should be detected, investigated and treated.

Few clinicians are aware of the high prevalence of pre-operative anaemia in patients scheduled to undergo surgery. Surgeons, anaesthetists and patients worry about postoperative complications, but how many are aware that a significant risk factor is pre-operative anaemia? Budget holders have little idea of the higher costs of healthcare in anaemic compared to non-anaemic patients who undergo surgery. Of all the physiological derangements that we might wish to optimise in surgical patients, treating anaemia before surgery is one of the easiest and yet it is infrequently done. The literature on pre-operative anaemia is limited, being a subject that has attracted only modest interest in anaesthesia and surgery. However, the common themes from several large observational studies are worrying and should already compel us to do much more about this important risk factor.

AAGBI Core Topics in Anaesthesia 2015, Edited by William Harrop-Griffiths, Richard Griffiths and Felicity Plaat.
© 2015 The Association of Anaesthetists of Great Britain and Ireland (AAGBI).
Published 2015 by John Wiley & Sons, Ltd.

Definitions of anaemia

What we mean by anaemia matters for diagnosis and treatment. In 1968, a World Health Organization (WHO) Scientific Group defined 'anaemia' as a haemoglobin concentration (Hb) of <12 g.l^{-1} in adult, non-pregnant females or <13 g.l^{-1} in adult males [1]. These cut-off values were derived from a small dataset, but the definition has stuck, and the definition is widely used in epidemiological studies. In clinical publications, anaemia can represent a variety of conditions. Sometimes the word is used generically, implying a very low Hb or haematocrit that the authors consider abnormal. Textbooks of haematology propose their own definitions, and laboratories across the country do not quote the same normal ranges for Hb. Clinicians refer to 'mild' or 'moderate' anaemia with no common understanding of not only when these adjectives should apply but also when the patient should be told if they are or they are not anaemic.

Prevalence

In the general population, the prevalence of anaemia depends on age, gender, pregnancy and the economic development of the country in which the population is being surveyed. Prevalences range in the elderly (men and women aged ≥60 years) from 12.2% in the most highly developed countries to 48.1% in the least developed [2]. The prevalence of pre-operative anaemia also varies, partly because several definitions are used. A figure of 20–40% is representative for major elective cardiac and non-cardiac surgery (Table 10.1).

Clinical implications of anaemia

A very low Hb will impair oxygen delivery. Studies in animals and humans suggest that 'critical oxygen delivery', the lowest oxygen delivery at which ischaemic sequelae are detectable, is around 7–10 mL O_2 min^{-1} kg^{-1}, which corresponds to Hb levels of 3–4 g.l^{-1} in humans. In healthy, conscious volunteers at rest, decreasing the Hb to 5 g.l^{-1} by isovolaemic haemodilution did not result in a decrease in oxygen consumption or an increase in lactate [3]. Compensatory mechanisms for anaemia include an increase in cardiac output, increased tissue oxygen extraction and alterations in microcirculatory blood flow.

How low must the Hb get before we see adverse postoperative outcomes? In a unique study that examined the natural history of surgical patients who did not accept a blood transfusion for religious reasons, Carson

Table 10.1 Studies in which the prevalence of pre-operative anaemia has been measured. Some of these studies are discussed in the text

Author (year of publication)	Years in which surgery was performed	Patient population	Country of study	Number of patients surveyed	Definition of anaemia	Prevalence of pre-operative anaemia
Goodnough (1992)	N/A	Elective orthopaedic surgery	USA	281	Hct ≤ 39%	26%
Rogers (2008)	5-year period before 2008	Elective hip arthroplasty	UK	322	Hb < 12.0 g.l^{-1}	9%
Greenky (2012)	2000–2007	Elective hip or knee arthroplasty	USA	15,722	WHO	20%
Kulier (2007)	1996–2000	Coronary artery bypass grafting	Worldwide	4,804	WHO	Male: 28% Female: 36%
Karkouti (2008)	2004	Cardiac surgery	Canada	3,500	Hb < 12.5 g.l^{-1}	26%
Dunne (2002)	1995–2000	Non-cardiac surgery	USA	6,301	Hct < 36%	34%
Wu (2007)	1997–2004	Major non-cardiac surgery in patients >65 years old	USA	310,311	Hct < 39%	43%
Beattie (2009)	2003–2006	Major non-cardiac surgery	Canada	7,759	WHO	Male: 40% Female: 40%
Leichtle (2011)	2005–2008	Elective open or laparoscopic colectomy	USA	23,348	Hct < 38%	47%
Musallam (2011)	2008	Major non-cardiac surgery	Worldwide	227,425	Hct < 36% female Hct < 39% male	30%

Hct, haematocrit.

et al. found an association between pre-operative Hb and postoperative mortality [4]. The lowest postoperative mortality was found in patients without cardiovascular disease, in those with the highest pre-operative Hb or those who experienced the lowest decrease in Hb after surgery. By comparison, the risk of death in patients with cardiovascular disease (angina, myocardial infarction, congestive heart failure or peripheral vascular disease) was 1.5 to 10 times higher as pre-operative Hb decreased to less than 12 g.l^{-1}. The odds ratio for postoperative mortality increased 16-fold as pre-operative Hb decreased from 12 to 6 g.l^{-1} in patients with cardiovascular disease, but barely doubled in patients without.

We may conclude that without blood transfusion the impact of a low pre-operative Hb on postoperative mortality depends on the Hb concentration at the start of surgery, presence or absence of cardiovascular disease, and the magnitude of the blood loss.

Pre-operative anaemia and postoperative outcome

Most of us think that pre-operative anaemia is a marker of the severity of the patient's illness. Given that assumption, observational studies are unhelpful because comparing outcomes of anaemic and non-anaemic patients would be just a surrogate for comparing sick patients with those who are less sick. In perhaps the earliest publication on pre-operative anaemia, Lunn and Elwood recognised this problem [5]. They obtained the Hb value at the start of surgery in 1,584 patients in Cardiff, and showed a significant association between the pre-operative Hb and in-hospital mortality. In their own words they concluded: ' . . . the hypothesis which best explains the association . . . is that pre-operative haemoglobin level reflects the severity of the underlying condition which has necessitated surgery. A randomised clinical trial would test the alternative hypothesis that anaemia constitutes an additional risk in surgical procedures'.

They therefore proposed a way to establish if pre-operative anaemia is in itself an important risk factor. However, in the intervening 45 years, such a randomised study has not been performed. One has to wonder whether this is because postoperative outcomes have improved so much in that time and pre-operative anaemia is no longer a concern, or simply because a totally effective treatment for anaemia already exists – blood transfusion.

Risk factors for peri-operative blood transfusion

Peri-operative transfusion is more likely if blood loss is marked. Centres that perform 'bloodless surgery' emphasise the importance of surgical

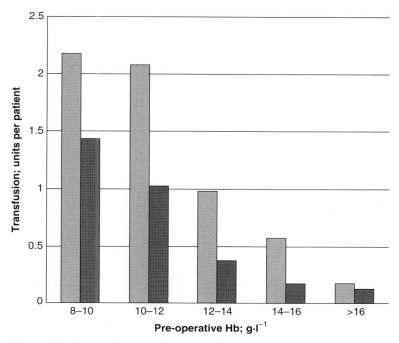

Figure 10.1 Transfusion rate is inversely related to pre-operative Hb. This example is taken from an audit of blood use in hip (left bar) and knee (right bar) replacement surgery [7].
Source: Taylor et al. 2005 [7]. Reproduced with permission of the authors.

techniques in minimising blood loss on the operating table. Although the skill of the surgeon, the conduct of the surgical team and the type of surgery are important considerations, one of the strongest predictors of peri-operative blood transfusion is the pre-operative Hb [6]. Pre-operative Hb and transfusion rate are negatively correlated as illustrated in Figure 10.1. This example was taken from an audit of blood use in orthopaedic surgery (867 hip and 883 knee replacements) in 13 hospitals [7]. In patients with a pre-operative Hb <12 g.l^{-1}, the transfusion rate was 77% for hip and 50% for knee surgery, compared with 37% and 15% respectively if the pre-operative Hb was >12 g.l^{-1}. A similar pattern will be seen in all types of surgery for which blood transfusion is usually required.

Risk factors for postoperative mortality and morbidity

The Veterans Health Administration (VHA) in the USA started to collect peri-operative data in the 1990s to audit surgical outcome. This initiative led to the establishment of the National Surgical Quality Improvement Program (VA-NSQIP) [8] and later the American College of Surgeons database for non-VHA hospitals (ACS-NSQIP). These programs provide an important source of prospectively collected national data on surgical outcomes.

Dunne et al. found that one-third of the 6301 patients who underwent non-cardiac surgery in the Maryland Healthcare system were anaemic (defined as a haematocrit <36%). These patients stayed in hospital longer and had higher rates of blood transfusion, postoperative pneumonia and death than non-anaemic patients [9].

In another study of 310,311 patients from 132 VHA hospitals, Wu et al. observed the lowest mortality in patients with haematocrit of 45–47.9% before surgery [10]. As the haematocrit decreased, mortality increased (from 1.7 to 26.7%), as did the rate of postoperative cardiac events (from 1% to 8.6%). A 1% decrease in the pre-operative haematocrit below 39% was accompanied by a 1.6% increase in postoperative mortality, but this relationship was not adjusted for blood transfusion.

These two studies show a troubling association between a low pre-operative Hb (haematocrit <36% or <39%) and adverse outcomes, but the questions that many of us would like to ask are: was the low Hb just an epiphenomenon and were adverse outcomes caused by blood transfusion or by low Hb concentration per se? In the absence of prospective, randomised, controlled trials of the sort that Lunn and Elwood suggested in 1970, we are left with other observational studies in which statistical methods have been used to adjust for peri-operative confounders and blood transfusion.

Pre-operative anaemia is an independent risk factor

In the first study that highlighted the risk of pre-operative anaemia in cardiac surgery, Kulier et al. found that pre-operative anaemia was an independent risk factor for non-cardiac complications: cerebral, renal, gastrointestinal, pulmonary and infective events (Figure 10.2) [11]. The data came from 4,804 patients undergoing coronary artery bypass grafting. In this cohort, 28.1% of male and 35.9% of female patients were anaemic before surgery, according to the WHO definition.

In 7,759 patients who underwent major non-cardiac surgery in a Toronto hospital, anaemic patients had a higher blood transfusion rate and twice the mortality of non-anaemic patients. The higher mortality was independent of blood transfusion (Figure 10.3) [12].

In 3,500 patients undergoing elective cardiac surgery, pre-operative anaemia (Hb <12.5 g.l^{-1}) was associated with a higher risk of in-hospital death, stroke and renal failure, independent of blood transfusion and

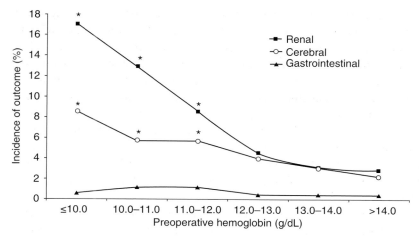

Figure 10.2 Lower pre-operative Hb in cardiac surgery is associated with a higher incidence of adverse renal and cerebral outcomes [11].
Source: Kulier et al. 2007 [11]. Reproduced with permission of Lippincott, Williams & Wilkins.

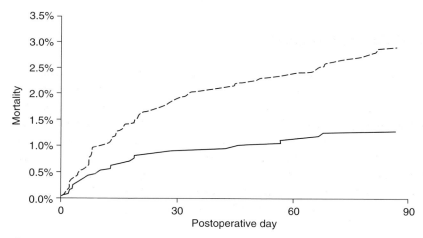

Figure 10.3 Time to event in risk (propensity) matched non-anaemic (solid line) and anaemic patients (broken line), showing a higher postoperative mortality in anaemic patients [12].
Source: Beattie et al. 2009 [12]. Reproduced with permission of Lippincott, Williams & Wilkins.

peri-operative confounders [13]. The data were pooled from seven Canadian hospitals in which the prevalence of pre-operative anaemia ranged from 22% to 30%

Mussallam et al. analysed the ACS-NSQIP data collected in 2008 [14]. Some 30% of the 227,425 patients were anaemic by WHO criteria. Anaemic patients were more likely to be elderly, to be in-patients at the time of surgery, and to have several comorbid conditions, giving them higher ASA physical status grades. As expected, the crude mortality rate in anaemic patients was higher than in non-anaemic patients but, after adjusting for confounders, pre-operative anaemia remained independently associated with increased mortality and morbidity. The independent risk of pre-operative anaemia was shown in all age groups, in both genders, and in all surgical specialties. While any of the comorbid conditions increased the likelihood of postoperative adverse outcomes, the presence of pre-operative anaemia augmented the impact of these comorbidities: an important and novel observation. Blood transfusion increased post-operative morbidity and mortality in both anaemic and non-anaemic patients.

We cannot ignore the fact that pre-operative anaemia is associated with higher rates of blood transfusion and increased postoperative morbidity and mortality. Although the data are observational, we can be persuaded that pre-operative anaemia is a risk factor for adverse postoperative outcomes and one that is probably independent of comorbidity and peri-operative blood transfusion.

Aetiology of anaemia

The commonest cause of anaemia worldwide is iron deficiency secondary to malnutrition or parasitic infestation. In developed countries, iron deficiency anaemia usually points to blood loss, resulting from gastrointestinal pathology or drugs, for example menstrual bleeding, malabsorption such as from coeliac disease, non-steroidal anti-inflammatory drugs and antiplatelet therapy. Anaemia is the commonest haematological disorder in the elderly and becomes more prevalent with increasing age. Causes of anaemia in the elderly include iron deficiency, anaemia of chronic disease, renal dysfunction and vitamin B12 or folate deficiency [15].

How should we manage the pre-operative patient with a low Hb?

Given what we know about the adverse consequences of pre-operative anaemia, we cannot continue to ignore it. There are already guidelines on treating pre-operative anaemia [16, 17], but little is known about the experience of institutions that implement them in their routine practice. The benefits of treating pre-operative anaemia should be demonstrated by enhanced short and long-term survival but these data are unavailable. For the clinician faced with the anaemic patient before elective surgery, the treatment goal is simple: increase the pre-operative Hb. A balance needs to be struck between attempting to increase the Hb without attention to the underlying aetiology of anaemia, and investigating the patient extensively to arrive at a diagnosis that may have no bearing on the surgery.

Patient assessment

Obtain a clinical history and enquire specifically, where relevant, about:
- Past episodes of anaemia or other blood disorders
- Blood donation
- Vegan or vegetarian diet
- Alcohol consumption
- Appetite
- Recent weight loss
- Symptoms of upper or lower gastrointestinal bleeding
- Change in bowel habit
- Menstrual bleeding
- Haematuria
- Concurrent medical conditions: arthritis, renal disease, malignancy or chronic infection
- Drugs: warfarin, antiplatelet and non-steroidal anti-inflammatory drugs

The history may identify the likely causes of anaemia and guide interpretation of laboratory tests. Referral to other specialists may form part of the evaluation, but this depends on whether the anaemia needs more invasive investigation or expert advice and management before the patient undergoes the planned surgery.

Investigations

All patients require an assessment of their iron status, renal and thyroid function. A C-reactive protein (CRP) level may be useful to detect the presence of an inflammatory state. Serum vitamin B12 and folate should be measured if the mean cell volume (MCV) shows macrocytosis (>100 fL).

Iron status

The most significant advance in our knowledge of iron physiology in the past decade relates to hepcidin, a small peptide secreted by the liver. Hepcidin is the regulatory hormone that controls iron release from enterocytes, hepatocytes and macrophages by binding to and inactivating the membrane receptor ferroportin. Hepcidin expression is stimulated by inflammation. Increased hepcidin decreases intestinal iron absorption and sequesters iron in storage sites, as occurs in anaemia of chronic disease (Figure 10.4) [18]. Iron overload suppresses hepcidin secretion. Techniques for the

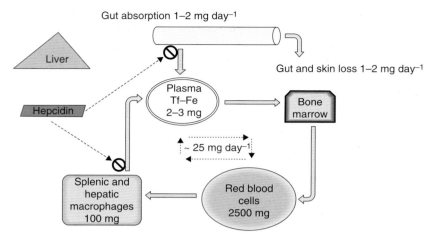

Figure 10.4 Most of the 3500–4000 mg of iron in the body is found in red blood cells and macrophages in the liver and spleen. The rest is present in iron-containing proteins such as myoglobin and cytochromes. Dietary iron intake of 1–2 mg per day is balanced by losses from the gut and desquamation. In the circulation, iron is bound to transferrin (Tf-Fe) and supplies the iron needed for erythropoiesis with about 25 mg recycled daily. Hepcidin expression in the liver is upregulated by inflammation. Hepcidin blocks iron absorption from the gut and sequesters iron in the macrophages by inactivating ferroportin at these sites, resulting in reduced iron availability for erythropoiesis.

measurement of hepcidin are evolving and one such is the futuristically named 'surface-enhanced laser desorption ionisation time-of-flight mass spectrometry'. Hepcidin may become a routine diagnostic test if its clinical utility can be demonstrated.

Iron stores

Ferritin is the ubiquitous intracellular protein that stores iron. In the circulation, ferritin is present at very low concentrations of around 50 μg L^{-1}. The amount of storage iron usually correlates with serum ferritin, which will be low in iron deficiency anaemia. Ferritin is an acute phase protein and serum levels increase in response to inflammation. Therefore, serum ferritin may be normal in some conditions, for example infection, malignancy, inflammatory bowel disease and rheumatoid arthritis, even when iron stores may be low. An elevated CRP might be a clue that a normal ferritin is the result of an acute phase response.

Iron supply

Iron is bound to transferrin in the circulation. Each molecule of transferrin binds two molecules of iron. Normally, 20–45% of the binding sites on transferrin are occupied by Fe^{3+} ions. Although transferrin-bound iron represents only 0.1% of the total body iron, this is the iron that is transferred from the gut, to and from storage sites, and supplied to the marrow for erythropoiesis. A transferrin saturation (TSAT) of <20% is a moderately sensitive indicator of iron deficiency. The NICE guideline for the management of chronic kidney disease advises that a TSAT <20% (and ferritin <100 µg L^{-1}) indicates absolute iron deficiency [19]. When the ferritin is not low, a TSAT <20% may indicate 'functional iron deficiency', in which the supply of iron to the marrow is limited despite adequate iron stores, probably as a consequence of elevated hepcidin, causing a state of iron-restricted erythropoiesis.

Some laboratories report total iron-binding capacity (TIBC) instead of TSAT. The TIBC is a test that measures the maximum amount of iron needed to totally saturate transferrin. Therefore, the TIBC is an indirect method of determining the amount of transferrin. Iron deficiency leads to increased serum transferrin, lower saturation of transferrin and consequently an increased TIBC. Serum iron level fluctuates throughout the day and should not be used to assess iron status.

Other tests

A common approach to the evaluation of anaemia is to subdivide the condition into microcytic, normocytic and macrocytic types according to the MCV. Most pre-operative patients with a low Hb tend to fall into the normocytic group, which should not be assumed to be synonymous with anaemia of chronic disease. Early iron deficiency anaemia presents as a normocytic anaemia. Erythrocytes become microcytic and hypochromic only at a very late stage of iron depletion.

The difficulty with differentiating anaemia due to inflammation, when ferritin is elevated, from anaemia of chronic disease with concurrent iron deficiency, highlights the need to assess iron status by other means. Alternative tests that have been scrutinised include plasma soluble transferrin receptor (sTfR), sTfR/log ferritin (sTfR index), percentage of hypochromic red cells and Hb content of reticulocytes [20]. All of these newer tests, some of which have been around for years, suffer from the problem that, singly or in combination, they do not offer the very high sensitivity and specificity desired of any diagnostic test.

Treatment of iron deficiency

Iron deficiency may be the commonest cause of anaemia in pre-operative patients. The decision to use oral or intravenous iron will be depend on the time available for treatment and whether oral iron is appropriate or tolerated.

Oral iron

Oral iron can be an effective treatment for iron deficiency anaemia if there is sufficient time, which is about 4 weeks for a response, if gut absorption is adequate, and if inflammatory conditions associated with elevated hepcidin can be excluded. However, some patients will develop side effects from oral iron, which are mostly gastrointestinal and which may be sufficiently bothersome that they will stop taking the tablets. Tolerance and efficacy might be improved if patients are given simple advice on when and how to take the tablets and are not prescribed the highest replacement dosage at the start of therapy. The recommended dose of elemental iron is 100–200 mg per day, but the maximum absorptive capacity of the duodenum reduces iron intake to no more than 10–20% of the dose ingested. It is impossible to be sure about compliance, and the only way to know if the treatment has worked is to repeat the Hb a few weeks later. Failure of oral iron therapy does not mean that the patient is not iron deficient. Although it is the standard first-line treatment for iron deficiency anaemia, oral iron is not the most effective.

Intravenous iron

Iron replacement can be achieved more reliably and rapidly if given intravenously. Intravenous iron preparations are iron-carbohydrate complexes and those currently available in the UK are summarised in Table 10.2. There is consensus that intravenous iron should be offered to patients who do not tolerate or respond to oral iron [21]. Patients with inflammatory bowel disease should not be given oral iron. Studies in several clinical settings have found that, compared to oral iron, treatment with intravenous iron results in a greater increase in Hb, higher levels of iron stores or both. Auerbach et al. have written an informative review on intravenous iron therapy [22].

Dose of intravenous iron

The dose of intravenous iron needed to treat iron deficiency anaemia can be estimated from the assumption that 10–15 mg kg^{-1} of iron is required to replenish the body's iron stores, and that 1 g of Hb contains 3.4 mg of iron.

Table 10.2 Intravenous iron formulations available in the UK in 2014

Trade name	Composition	Maximum single dose	Approximate cost per 1000 mg*
Cosmofer	Iron dextran	20 mg kg^{-1}	£ 79
Ferinject	Ferric carboxymaltose	1000 mg (not exceeding 15 mg kg^{-1})	£191
Monofer	Iron isomaltoside	20 mg kg^{-1}	£169
Venofer	Iron sucrose	200 mg	£ 93

*Based on prices quoted in British National Formulary.

The Ganzoni equation is the standard formula that is used to calculate the replacement dose:

$$\text{Iron dose (mg)} = \text{body weight (kg)} \times [\text{target Hb} - \text{actual Hb (g.l}^{-1})]$$
$$\times 2.4 + \text{iron stores (mg)}$$

In practice, most pre-operative patients will need around 1000 mg of intravenous iron, which can be given as a single infusion. Blood loss of 500 mL in a non-anaemic individual (assuming Hb = 14.0 g.l^{-1}) is equivalent to a loss of about 250 mg of iron.

Safety and efficacy of intravenous iron

Intravenous iron is stigmatised. Older clinicians may remember parenteral iron as a painful intramuscular injection, while many clinicians believe it is a hazardous infusion with the potential to precipitate anaphylactic shock. In the author's own hospital, it was decreed several years ago that intravenous adrenaline, hydrocortisone and chlorpheniramine have to be prescribed alongside intravenous iron, and the infusion has to be given in a location in which a doctor and cardiac defibrillator are immediately available. Serious adverse reactions can occur with intravenous iron, but they are exceedingly rare and perhaps even less likely with the latest formulations.

All parenteral iron preparations are effective for iron replacement, and the key difference between them, apart from cost, comes down to whether the iron deficit can be replaced in one go ('total dose infusion'), which makes for a convenient strategy when treating outpatients (see Table 10.2). A decade ago, intravenous iron was used almost exclusively in patients on haemodialysis. Today, there are many more clinical settings: iron deficiency anaemia, chemotherapy-induced anaemia, pregnancy, peri-operative anaemia and heart failure, in which intravenous iron has been investigated and used to treat or exclude iron deficiency.

Erythropoietin

In the UK, the only erythropoiesis-stimulating agent licensed specifically for pre-operative anaemia is epoetin alfa, a recombinant human erythropoietin. One recommended dosing scheme is 600 units kg^{-1} given at weekly intervals 3 weeks before surgery, with a fourth dose on the day of surgery. There is little doubt that intravenous iron combined with an erythropoiesis-stimulating agent can be more effective than intravenous iron alone at increasing the Hb. In healthy volunteers subjected to phlebotomy, the level of endogenous erythropoietin was higher after blood loss but remained within the normal range. Associated with this, maximal erythropoiesis increased the mass of red cells by around 20% after even a moderate amount of blood was removed. Administration of an erythropoiesis-stimulating agent enhanced the response in a dose-dependent fashion, with an increase in red cells of 30% at lower doses and up to 80% at higher doses of the erythropoiesis-stimulating agent [23]. Using an erythropoiesis-stimulating agent may not be essential to treat anaemia but it should not surprise us that its addition enhances erythropoiesis. The clue is in the name. The practical problem of using epoetin is the need to give at least three doses before surgery. All erythropoiesis-stimulating agents share the same biological properties. Darbepoetin, a longer-acting agent, may be a more convenient alternative, but it is not licensed for the treatment of pre-operative anaemia.

Treatment of coexisting pathologies

Renal disease
The subject of chronic kidney disease and anaemia warrants at least an entire chapter, if not an entire book. The degree of renal impairment should be categorised using the calculated glomerular filtration rate (GFR) on a scale consistent with internationally agreed definitions, and not simply by inferring from the creatinine value [24]. Inadequate erythropoietin secretion by the kidney may not become a risk factor for anaemia until the GFR is at least 60 mL min^{-1} per 1.73 m^2 and probably much lower [25]. At any level of renal dysfunction, the first priority in the evaluation of anaemia remains the identification and treatment of iron deficiency and other reversible causes. A substantial proportion of anaemic patients with impaired renal function will be iron deficient.

Vitamin B12 and folate deficiency
It is standard practice to measure vitamin B12 and folate levels in the work up of any anaemic patient. However, this approach may need to be challenged. In a general population of very elderly (≥85 years) persons, who should have the highest prevalence of anaemia, there was no difference in Hb between those with or without B12 deficiency. In a subsequent follow up over 5 years, there was no association between vitamin B12 deficiency and the development of anaemia. A large survey of elderly outpatients could not find an association between vitamin B12 or folate levels and anaemia [26, 27]. Faced with these data, a pragmatic solution is to follow the NICE 'do not do' recommendation, which states: 'tests for vitamin B12 and folate deficiency in adults should not be carried out unless a full blood count and mean red cell volume show macrocytosis' [28].

Other aetiologies
Thyroid hormones stimulate erythropoiesis, and anaemia is more likely to accompany hypothyroidism than hyperthyroidism. Symptoms of hypothyroidism may not be clinically apparent, and thyroid function tests might be the only way in which the diagnosis is made. Hyperthyroid and

overtly hypothyroid patients are at increased risk of peri-operative complications, and elective surgery may have to be re-scheduled, if for no other reason than to correct thyroid dysfunction.

The aetiology of anaemia cannot be easily determined in a proportion of patients owing to the limited specificity of our conventional screening tests [29]. Bone marrow suppression such as early myelodysplasia, impaired release of or response to endogenous erythropoietin, or drug interactions impairing iron absorption or erythropoiesis, for example with antacids, proton-pump inhibitors and angiotensin-converting enzyme inhibitors, may account for anaemia in some patients. Therefore, despite a comprehensive investigation, one should expect to meet some patients in whom the aetiology of anaemia is uncertain and a logical treatment cannot be proposed.

In summary, the management of pre-operative anaemia will require:
- Recognition of a low Hb
- Clinical history
- Routine investigations to assess iron status, renal and thyroid function
- Treatment, usually of iron deficiency in the majority of patients
- Referral to specialists for further investigation, for a minority, if the diagnosis of anaemia is more urgent than surgery

With good organisation of the pre-operative assessment process, most patients can and should be treated without the need to postpone surgery.

Quality assurance

The efficacy of treating pre-operative anaemia must be measured by recording, at the very least, pre-treatment and post-treatment Hb, the time interval between treatment and surgery, the peri-operative use of blood products, length of hospital stay, major complications and mortality. An estimate of the incidence and type of treatment side effects is essential. If comparison can be made with historical or other control data, any benefit of the intervention will be easier to see and can be used to support a business case – so necessary in modern healthcare – for continuing or extending the rationale for treating pre-operative anaemia. At least two prospective, randomised, controlled trials are ongoing in the UK to assess the impact of treating a low pre-operative Hb in cardiac and in open abdominal surgery.

Conclusions

The patient who is anaemic before surgery should be worried. Can clinicians overcome the therapeutic nihilism that has been the norm for pre-operative anaemia? We must recognise the condition for what it is: a risk factor that increases postoperative complications and the likelihood of death, a comorbidity that is largely reversible and, in most cases, a simple diagnosis that if left untreated will predictably lead to expensive and adverse consequences.

Declaration of interests

The author is chief investigator of a prospective, randomised, controlled trial of the treatment of low pre-operative Hb in cardiac surgery. The study is partly funded by Pharmacosmos A/S (Denmark), manufacturer of the intravenous iron agents Cosmofer® and Monofer®.

References

1. Beutler E, Waalen J. The definition of anemia: what is the lower limit of normal of the blood hemoglobin concentration? *Blood* 2006; **107**: 1747–1750.
2. McLean E, Cogswell M, Egli I, Wojdyla D, de Benoist B. Worldwide prevalence of anaemia, WHO vitamin and mineral nutrition information system, 1993-2005. *Public Health Nutrition* 2009; **12**: 444–454.
3. Weiskopf RB, Viele MK, Feiner J, et al. Human cardiovascular and metabolic response to acute, severe isovolemic anemia. *Journal of the Americal Medical Association* 1998; **279**: 217–221.
4. Carson J, Duff A, Poses R, et al. Effect of anaemia and cardiovascular disease on surgical mortality and morbidity. *Lancet* 1996; **348**: 1055–1060.
5. Lunn JN, Elwood PC. Anaemia and surgery. *British Medical Journal* 1970; **3**: 71–73.
6. The Society of Thoracic Surgeons Blood Conservation Guideline Task Force. Ferraris VA, Ferraris SP, et al. Perioperative blood transfusion and blood conservation in cardiac surgery: The society of thoracic surgeons and the society of cardiovascular anesthesiologists clinical practice guideline. *Annals of Thoracic Surgery* 2007; **83**: S27–S86.
7. Taylor C, Best A, Lumley M, Hartley J, Baker C, Pailing M. Audit of blood use in orthopaedic surgery - comparative report. March 2005. West Midlands Regional Transfusion Committee. www.transfusionguidelines.org.uk/uk-transfusion-committees/regional-transfusion-committees/audits/audits/audit-of-blood-use-in-orthopaedic-surgery-march-2005/download-file/rtc-wmids_audit_hip_and_knee .pdf (accessed 29/12/2014).
8. Khuri SF, Daley J, Henderson W, et al. The Department of Veterans Affairs' NSQIP: the first national, validated, outcome-based, risk-adjusted, and peer-controlled program for the measurement and enhancement of the quality of surgical care. National VA surgical quality improvement program. *Annals of Surgery* 1998; **228**: 491–507.
9. Dunne JR, Malone D, Tracy JK, Gannon C, Napolitano LM. Perioperative anemia: an independent risk factor for infection, mortality, and resource utilization in surgery. *Journal of Surgical Research* 2002; **102**: 237–244.
10. Wu W-C, Schifftner TL, Henderson WG, et al. Preoperative hematocrit levels and postoperative outcomes in older patients undergoing noncardiac surgery. *Journal of the American Medical Association* 2007; **297**: 2481–2488.
11. Kulier A, Levin J, Moser R, et al. Impact of preoperative anemia on outcome in patients undergoing coronary artery bypass graft surgery. *Circulation* 2007; **116**: 471–479.
12. Beattie WS, Karkouti K, Wijeysundera DN, Tait G. Risk associated with preoperative

anemia in noncardiac surgery: a single-center cohort study. *Anesthesiology* 2009; **110**: 574–581.

13. Karkouti K, Wijeysundera DN, Beattie WS. Risk associated with preoperative anemia in cardiac surgery: a multicenter cohort study. *Circulation* 2008; **117**: 478–484.

14. Musallam KM, Tamim HM, Richards T, et al. Preoperative anaemia and postoperative outcomes in non-cardiac surgery: a retrospective cohort study. *Lancet* 2011; **378**: 1396–1407.

15. Guralnik JM, Eisenstaedt RS, Ferrucci L, Klein HG, Woodman RC. Prevalence of anemia in persons 65 years and older in the United States: evidence for a high rate of unexplained anemia. *Blood* 2004; **104**: 2263–2268.

16. Goodnough LT, Shander A, Spivak JL, et al. Detection, evaluation, and management of anemia in the elective surgical patient. *Anesthesia & Analgesia* 2005; **101**: 1858–1861.

17. Goodnough LT, Maniatis A, Earnshaw P, et al. Detection, evaluation, and management of preoperative anaemia in the elective orthopaedic surgical patient: NATA guidelines. *British Journal of Anaesthesia* 2011; **106**: 13–22.

18. Ganz T Hepcidin and iron regulation, 10 years later. *Blood* 2011; **117**: 4425–4433.

19. Anaemia management in people with chronic kidney disease. NICE clinical guideline 114: National Institute for Health and Care Excellence, 2011.

20. Wish JB. Assessing iron status: beyond serum ferritin and transferrin saturation. *Clinical Journal of the American Society of Nephrology* 2006; **1**: S4–S8.

21. Beris P, Muñoz M, Garcia-Erce JA, Thomas D, Maniatis A, Van der Linden P. Perioperative anaemia management: consensus statement on the role of intravenous iron. *British Journal of Anaesthesia* 2008; **100**: 599–604.

22. Auerbach M, Coyne D, Ballard H. Intravenous iron: from anathema to standard of care. *American Journal of Hematology* 2008; **83**: 580–588.

23. Goodnough LT, Skikne B, Brugnara C. Erythropoietin, iron, and erythropoiesis. *Blood* 2000; **96**: 823–833.

24. KDIGO 2012 Clinical Practice Guideline For The Evaluation And Management Of Chronic Kidney Disease. *Kidney International Supplements* 2013; **3.** http://www.kdigo. org/clinical_practice_guidelines/pdf/CKD/KDIGO_2012_CKD_GL.pdf (accessed 29/12/2014).

25. Ble A, Fink JC, Woodman RC, et al. Renal function, erythropoietin, and anemia of older persons: the InCHIANTI Study. *Archives of Internal Medicine* 2005; **165**: 2222–2227.

26. den Elzen WP, Westendorp RG, Frölich M, de Ruijter W, Assendelft WJ, Gussekloo J. Vitamin B12 and folate and the risk of anemia in old age: the Leiden 85-Plus Study. *Archives of Internal Medicine* 2008; **168**: 2238–2244.

27. Lippi G, Montagnana M, Targher G, Guidi GC. Vitamin B12, folate, and anemia in old age. *Archives of Internal Medicine* 2009; **169**: 716.

28. NICE. Do not do recommendation. http://bit.ly/1ulOD2v (accessed 21/1/2015).

29. Guralnik JM, Ershler WB, Schrier SL, Picozzi VJ. Anemia in the elderly: a public health crisis in hematology. *Hematology* 2005; **2005**: 528–532.

30. Rogers BA, Cowie A, Alcock C, Rosson JW. Identification and treatment of anaemia in patients awaiting hip replacement. *Annals of the Royal College of Surgeons of England* 2008; **90**: 504–507.

31. Greenky M, Gandhi K, Pulido L, Restrepo C, Parvizi J. Preoperative anemia in total joint arthroplasty: is it associated with periprosthetic joint infection? *Clinical Orthopaedics and Related Research* 2012; **470**: 2695–2701.

32. Leichtle SW, Mouawad NJ, Lampman R, Singal B, Cleary RK. Does preoperative anemia adversely affect colon and rectal surgery outcomes? *Journal of the American College of Surgeons* 2011; **212**: 187–194.